MMM THEORY

A New Paradigm in Medicine

THE INFLAMMATION TREATMENT BOOK:
REVEALING THE ROOT CAUSE OF DISEASE,
ITS PREVENTION & TREATMENT

Dr. Chris D. Meletis

Howard M. Simon

MMM THEORY

A New Paradigm in Medicine

The inflammation treatment book: revealing the root cause of disease, its prevention & treatment

Dr. Chris D. Meletis & Howard M. Simon

My friend, Professor Bruce Ames, PhD, has such a reverence for the human body and biochemistry. He taught me to ask questions such as "Why would the body attack itself?" MMM Theory attempts to answer that question.

- H.M.S.

TABLE OF CONTENTS

DISCLAIMER

This book is intended to supplement, not replace, the advice of a trained health professional. If you know or suspect that you have a health problem, you should consult a health professional. The authors and publisher specifically disclaim any liability, loss, or risk, personal or otherwise, that is incurred as a consequence, directly or indirectly, of the use and application of any of the contents of this book.

The information and any nutritional supplements mentioned in this book have not been evaluated by the Food and Drug Administration. The information and products mentioned herein are not intended to diagnose, treat, cure, or prevent any disease.

CHAPTER ONE

MMM THEORY - OVERVIEW OF THE NEW MEDICAL PARADIGM

Introduction to MMM Theory

This book and the Microbial Mucosal Milieu theory result from my many years of suffering from Inflammatory Bowel Disease (IBD). Revelations, research, personal experimentation, and limited case studies led me to conceptualize an alternative understanding of my "disease" and many other conditions also categorized as "autoimmune disease."

The best way to read this book is to let go of everything you have learned about human or veterinary physiology and medicine. Since we know that you 'can't do this (and neither could I), I invite all scientists and doctors reading this book to use your knowledge and experience to challenge what you are reading and what you believe you know. We will help you integrate these new revelations throughout the book.

Here are a few definitions and concepts to help you understand our perspective or paradigm. It is likely different than what you have ever heard before but hopefully will explain concepts that you have wondered about for a long time.

The Microbial Mucosal Milieu—MMM for short—is an entity that exists throughout your entire body but is most visible and studied where it resides on the surface of your gastrointestinal tract – your mouth, throat, stomach, small intestines, bowel, and anus.

We have coined the new term Microbial Mucosal Milieu. MMM represents more than the three words used separately, just like saltwater may define an ecosystem, far beyond the simple definition of salt dissolved in water. The goal of this book is to explain MMM Theory, and yet, we have already identified additional chapters for book 2.

The MMM exists in and around every organ, system, and possibly every cell and organelle in the human or animal body. There is no barrier in the body, from the oral to the blood-brain barrier, to the lymph system, to individual cellular barriers that are not protected and served by the MMM.

There are about 10 times as many microbes as human cells in the human body. Thus, the MMM contains nearly 3.3 million genes compared to about 23,000 identified in the human body.

Current paradigms in medicine and medical tools do not easily enable identification of the MMM on other than external surfaces of the body, nor do they allow doctors to view functioning of the MMM.

The MMM regulates everything (nutrients, toxins, contaminants, waste) that enters the body and all organs, systems, and cells. It simultaneously regulates everything (cellular waste, toxins, contaminants) that is excreted by the body.

Imagine if your hot and cold water, sewage, electricity, heating, and cooling were all running through the same pipe in your house. What an immensely sophisticated adaptive system it would take to manage these flows simultaneously through the same pipe. I'm thinking of these as an analogy for your vascular, lymph, sinus, and gastrointestinal systems when I ask you to imagine beyond current dogma. Each of these body systems transport both nutrients and waste simultaneously through the same "pipe."

Computer engineers dealt with this issue in a two-dimensional model. They had to move information from one computer to another. This evolved into the internet, where packets of information move bidirectionally on the same wire, then via light on fiber-optic channels. As technology progressed, it became faster and far more complex, managing integration of hardwire networks, broadcast networks such as Wi-Fi, dealing with different speeds of communication and delays in delivery, switching between communication centers, text, images, and sound, integrating chef Emeril 'Lagasse's smellivision, and far more.

We are also just in our infancy of understanding how our body systems transport, and our microbiome propagates beneficial bacteria throughout our entire body in a complex fashion in yet-to-be understood pathways.

The accelerated growth of EMFs (electromagnetic field) emissions confounds our understanding of the MMM and its impact on health. EMFs could harm bacteria directly with heat or they could interfere with cellular, bacterial, and interspecies communications in ways not yet known. This will be discussed in later chapters.

Many diseases, such as autoimmune diseases, and diseases that have inflammation as a symptom are the body's response to microcontaminants in the organelle, cell, organ, or system. In the case of autoimmune diseases, we will show that the body is attacking the microcontaminants that have entered the organ or system, not attacking the body itself. So, we believe the term autoimmune is a misinterpretation of the physiology of the body's response. Contaminants are not diseases. However, our medical tools identify the collateral damage and interpret autoimmune diseases as the body attacking itself rather than attacking the microcontaminants that are "hidden" there.

My interpretation of autoimmune disease started with a realization of what was occurring in my gastrointestinal tract (GIT) and expanded as I discovered how similar other organs and systems in the body function. For many, this is an easy progression to understand, and thus we present the gastrointestinal tract as a focus, but it is only the beginning of our exploration of how our MMM works synergistically with the body. For the GIT offers the most visible example of the MMM at work or in a dysfunctional state using "modern" medical paradigm, tools and methods.

We have not yet decided if the body is the host or the superstructure for the MMM. This is perhaps an issue of the human ego – can we be anything other than the center of our own universe? Or put another way, who serves whom?

By regulating entry and exit throughout the body, the MMM has the ability to avoid, minimize, reduce, or stop the body's attack on microcontaminants in systems and organs.

The MMM provides a coordinated response to the environment and all parts of the body. Science now identifies this as undefined pathways of communication. MMM Theory says that is the MMM at work.

By regulating all pathways in the human body, the MMM has the potential to manage systemic body activities, leading to wellness and disease.

Aging, and diseases of aging, reflect episodic and long-term nutrient deficiency or depletion and accumulation of microcontaminants and waste in the body, and the growing body burden of that combination of factors according to Triage Theory developed by Professor Emeritus Bruce Ames, PhD.[15,16] Diseases of childhood represent an early susceptibility and accumulation of microcontaminants that the developing body is not strong enough to adapt to, and manifest as developmental diseases. The MMM plays a critical role in nutrient delivery, waste removal and microcontaminant accumulation.

There are so many new discoveries being made of never-before-seen systems in the body. They all support MMM theory of health and aging. These include the glymphatic system, the vascular system in bones, and the bacterial milieu in a woman's placenta. The placenta microbiome, identified about 10 years ago, changes the dogma that babies are sterile until birth.

Highlights of MMM Theory

We have several ways to share this new paradigm in medicine that I call MMM Theory. Our goal was to find a way for you to understand the limits of conventional thinking, opening your mind to a new paradigm.

Some people who read this book will be scientists and clinicians. Some will be health researchers, looking for new paths to explore, and some will be folks with a disease that just can't be explained or fully treated with conventional medicine. These people see that modern medicine can treat their symptoms, and this is helpful, but they are frustrated that doctors don't know the root cause of their problem, and therefore allopathic medicine's goal is remission of symptoms, rather than cure.

The hypothesis and treatments are relatively simple, but so new and profound, that it takes some thought and convincing for even an open-minded person to buy into it.

Here were our options for presenting our hypothesis, the supporting research, and the effect on various diseases and conditions.

1. Tell the story as a progression of the way the paradigm unfolded for me.
2. Start at the end, being the disease and its treatment, and work backward into the theory.
3. Present in-depth research and our alternative interpretation and conclusions that the research supports.
4. Start with the most profound concepts and explore how they impact various diseases and treatments later in the book.

We chose option 4.

Here is the briefest summary of what you will learn in this book.

The MMM exists throughout the body, in every organ, system, and cell in the body.

A healthy MMM protects your body from contaminants – both entering your body and entering any and every organ and system in your body.

The MMM consists of an evolving balance of beneficial and harmful bacteria, nutrients for the bacteria, and nutrients to enhance communication of the MMM with tissue, cells, and mitochondria in the body.

A contaminant is something that doesn't belong in your body such as air and water pollution. But it can also be something that belongs somewhere else in your body, such as hydrochloric acid which only belongs in your stomach.

The MMM is both resilient and fragile and can be damaged by antibiotics, anti-microbials, such as alcohol, hydrocarbons, pesticides, herbicides, cleaning chemicals, chlorine, heavy metals, plastic chemicals, radiation – such as 5G, a poor diet, and more toxins.

Damage to the MMM will allow contaminants to enter your body and your organs. Genetic susceptibility and physical injury will allow these contaminants to accumulate in your weakest system. This is a primary cause of disease.

Contaminants that enter a baby's brain contribute to diseases of childhood development. Contaminants that accumulate over a lifetime may cause or at least contribute to diseases of aging. Contaminants that accumulate in your mitochondria cause a lack of energy, stamina, and healing power.

The easiest place to explore the MMM is in the gastrointestinal tract – mouth, intestines, bowel - and on the skin. Very limited, and often misleading, conclusions can be drawn from thinking that the MMM exists only in places we can see, even with the best medical tools.

Current medical tools do not show molecules within a cell, such as a microcontaminant. Thus, science does not know they are there. But the MMM does "see" this and goes to work, sight unseen by humans, to protect the body from these contaminants.

Many diseases, including all diseases categorized as autoimmune disease, are not merely the body attacking itself. They reflect the body attacking contaminant-impacted areas. Like with a bee sting, the whole area becomes inflamed, not just the bee venom.

Speaking of inflammation, inflammation reflects the body's natural response to microcontaminants and other processes. Many diseases with inflammation as a symptom are initiated or potentiated by microcontaminants in the body.

The U.S. National Institutes of Health, National Institute of Environmental Health and Science (NIH, NIEHS) says inflammation is associated with diseases such as the following:[1]

- Autoimmune diseases like rheumatoid arthritis, colitis, and lupus
- Cardiovascular diseases like high blood pressure and heart disease
- Gastrointestinal disorders like inflammatory bowel disease
- Lung diseases like asthma
- Mental illnesses like depression
- Metabolic diseases like Type 2 diabetes
- Neurodegenerative diseases like 'Parkinson's disease
- Some types of cancer, like colon cancer

Microcontaminants lingering in the body and eliciting an immune response reflect mismanagement of the flow of nutrients and waste.

The MMM facilitates movement of nutrients and cellular waste to and from every cell in the body. This movement includes movement of the MMM itself. Approximately half of feces is MMM that have given their lives in the cause of supporting your body.

The MMM circulates throughout the body and manages circulation in multiple systems – such as blood, lymph, and intracellular spaces. This is where we developed our tube analogy. Imagine that your home had one pipe like your gastrointestinal tract or lymph system. Inside that pipe in your home, all mixed together, are clean hot and cold water, electricity, natural or propane gas, and wastewater from your sinks, showers, and toilets. **The MMM is so sophisticated that it can deliver and remove the appropriate inputs and outputs (nutrients and waste) which coexist in your blood, lymphatic, and sinuses, to the places where they are needed or excreted.**

For example, it is understood that many vitamins are generally absorbed into blood circulation in the large intestine. Yet we also know that the large intestine ferments nutrients and accumulates waste which is passed as fecal matter. So how does the body differentiate between nutrients that are being drawn from bolus in your colon and fecal matter which will be expelled?

If the body cannot remove microcontaminants from your cells, it will try to isolate them. The most effective way to isolate them is by storing them in fat. You know what happens when you store excess fat in your body. Here is a primary reason.

These microcontaminants may come from an external source, such as herbicides in food, heavy metals in water, hydrocarbons in smog, trace pharmaceutical drugs, or plastics in all these sources.

Bacterial diversity, proper nourishment, dietary diversity, avoiding MMM poisons, and balance are key to a healthy MMM. Chapter 9 will describe how to maintain and restore a healthy MMM.

Cardiologist Stephen Sinatra MD believed that the root cause of heart disease is inflammation. We say the root cause of inflammation is the MMM not operating at its best. This infers that the root cause of heart disease is a dysfunctional MMM.

Gastroenterologists, when asked, cannot pinpoint the root cause of GI diseases such as IBS, IBD, UC, etc. MMM theory posits that a weak MMM allows microcontaminants to damage the GI tract causing all these diseases.

Neurologists and researchers David Perlmutter MD and Aristo Vojdani PhD identify microcontaminants as a cause of brain and neurological diseases. MMM theory identifies a weakened MMM as the gatekeeper that allows these contaminants to cross the Blood Brain Barrier (BBB). Contaminants may also enter the neurological system through a specialized part of the lymph system, named the glymphatic system, which delivers nutrients and removes waste from the neurological system during sleep.

Or a weakened MMM does not properly facilitate passage of waste material, including senescent cells, out of the cell, brain, or neurological system. Imagine if you didn't take out just one bag of garbage from your house monthly, but it let it accumulate for years. In the body, this leads to diseases of aging.

HIGHLIGHTS

We have now posited the cause of inflammation. We will establish the cause of acute and chronic diseases and how to prevent the causes of inflammation. MMM Theory will thus show how to prevent and treat acute and chronic diseases that present as inflammatory diseases by supporting the MMM throughout the body.

Many conventional medical treatments that reduce symptoms may continue to be used in conjunction with resolving the underlying cause of inflammation and "disease." One just needs to be aware when they are treating the body's protective mechanisms.

Form, Fit and Function of the Microbial Mucosal Milieu

The topic of a healthy mucosal milieu—in my case, the gastrointestinal tract—has been the inspiration for my quest to pull together the scientific literature to support my health and wellness journey. You can use my knowledge to further your own quest for vibrant, good health.

As other medical conditions revealed their similarities to me during my research, and considering how many other individuals are experiencing the ravages of a disordered GI tract or a global disharmonious microbial-mucosal milieu, I have expanded my hypothesis to all organs, systems, and many diseases.

There is no argument that our body constantly speaks to us, with signs and symptoms of happiness, neutrality, or disharmony. There is a saying that captures the likelihood of our developing any number of health conditions: "Genetics predisposes, yet diet and lifestyle ultimately manifests." Yes, for scientists with a genetic focus there are instances where a condition is passed down from a parent to a child, known as autosomal dominant conditions. Yet, it can be argued that diet and lifestyle also impact these types of genetic disorders.

What is the Microbial Mucosal Milieu?

The microbial mucosal milieu (MMM) is an entity that is located throughout the body and is not limited to any particular location in the body. The microbial-mucosal milieu can be viewed as a continuously vacillating system that shifts with ongoing adaptation to maintain health-promoting homeostasis for both itself and the human body. Imagine for a moment the peak of a sand dune amid an expansive desert. The peak of that dune will have an ever-changing GPS location, just as homeostasis is always adapting and ever-changing.

Indeed, the MMM is characterized by localized microbial diversity, the surrounding microbiome, and genetics of each host. These characteristics manifest and vary throughout the entire body, not merely the gastrointestinal tract. Microbial diversity refers to the different kinds of bacteria you have in your body. The microbiome is the collection of good and bad bacteria, viruses, and fungi that live in your body. You can think of the MMM as a community or system. The vitality and robustness of the MMM depends upon the organism's health, nuclear genetics, mitochondrial function, food/nutrient supply or diet, physiological and psychological stresses, toxic burden, microbial exposure, and other epigenetic factors that we will explore in the chapters to come.

One of my favorite analogies to the concept of an MMM are the Star Trek TV shows and movies. Gene Roddenberry had great foresight, or good fortune of having great writers, imagining the human MMM, and showing how it works on Star Trek. Recall many scenes where Scotty says "Capt'n, (deflector) shields are up." And Captain Kirk orders the crew to fire phasers and photon torpedos! The shields act as an intelligent, semi-permeable membrane that protects the starship Enterprise, while allowing weapons to fire through them. On the other hand, the shields had to be manipulated or adapted to allow people to be transported bidirectionally through them.

What Is Epigenetics?

Epigenetics refers to the way lifestyle factors, behavior, and the environment impact the function of your genes. Unlike genetic changes, epigenetic alterations can be reversed. Epigenetic changes don't alter your DNA sequence, but they can influence how your body reads your DNA. They act like a switch that can turn genes on and off. Epigenetic changes can be passed on from mother to child and even to grandchildren.

Over time, the MMM, like the peak of the proverbial sand dune, fluctuates on a scale from thriving to surviving to disease (cellular disharmony).

The MMM is more than the sum of its components - the microbiota, microbiome, mucosa, or metabolome (the metabolites produced by cells during metabolism). The MMM is the composite entity that serves as the aggregate modulator of whole-body health.

MMM Intelligence

The adaptive intelligence of the MMM cannot be well comprehended or underestimated.

Ray Bradbury in his short story *Here There Be Tygers*, first published in 1951, makes a great case for appreciating intelligence in objects that we do not normally attribute intelligence to. The story presents a rocket expedition seeking to mine resources for Earth, lured to a planet to see whether its natural resources can be harvested for the human race. The explorers discover a paradise which seems to provide for them whatever they desire even as they think of it. One crew member wants to mine the planet for all that they can gain. The other crew members realize that the planet is alive, has female characteristics, and only wants the male explorers to stay and enjoy the love that the planet bestows on them. One explorer stays and the others leave and report the planet as hostile, so as to protect its hidden beauty.

The MMM regulates everything (nutrients, toxins, contaminants, waste) that enters the body and individually enters and leaves all organs, systems, and cells in the body. It simultaneously regulates everything (cellular waste, toxins, contaminants) that are excreted by the body.

Just as I asked you to imagine if your hot and cold water, your sewage, electricity, heating and cooling were all running through the same pipe in your house, I ask you to imagine two of the three main flows – your lymph and gastrointestinal systems –

throughout your body in the same way. What an immensely sophisticated adaptive system it would take to manage these flows simultaneously through the same pipe.

Specifically, both your gastrointestinal tract and your lymph systems carry nourishment (water and nutrients), cellular waste, oxygen and carbon dioxide essentially in the same tube. There is no point of demarcation where the tube stops carrying nutrients and starts carrying waste. We will delve into this further when we ask the questions: What is sanitary? How are nutrients and waste selectively removed from the flows? What causes mismanagement of the flows? What is the effect of mismanagement of the flows?

Building a Healthy Ecology for a Thriving MMM

MMM Theory will show that it does matter what building blocks we provide our body and the MMM. There is a consequence and truth to the adage "We are what we eat from our head to our feet." But wait, there is more to the story. Are we merely feeding ourselves? The answer is a resounding no!

The next time you place a delicious morsel in your mouth, you are fueling the cells of your body and the energy production to sustain life. You are also feeding the microbial community that lives throughout your body but is usually only thought of as populating your GI tract. This microbial community ultimately impacts all organs and tissues of your body. The integrity of the mucosal lining of your GI tract that serves as the gut homeland security system will, directly and indirectly, be impacted by that morsel of food. There will be a ripple effect as it nurtures your GI microbes so they can properly sustain a healthy microbiome or alter essential short-chain fatty acids such as butyrate.

No Longer in Kansas

Like Dorothy in *The Wizard of Oz* proclaimed, "Toto, I've a feeling we're not in Kansas anymore."

We now live in a world of toxins, electromagnetic fields (EMFs), pesticides, herbicides, genetically modified foods, microwave-modified foods, processed food galore, concentrated human pollutants, heavy metals, plastics, xenoestrogens (natural or synthetic compounds that mirror the effects of estrogen produced in the body or that trigger estrogen production), and countless medications—whether prescribed or in your water supply—that alter the microbial and mucosal health of the body.

Over 70 percent of the "food products" sold in the local supermarket did not exist a generation ago. Thus, we nourish current and future generations with untested and questionable building materials. Potentially equally as important is that we are feeding the microbiota that has co-existed with humanity over the generations with toxins and "foodstuffs." This ultimately impacts the microbiota's ability to participate optimally in the symbiotic relationship with us, the host. Finally, how we fuel and treat our bodies affects their ecology and ability to thrive, with a well-noted ripple effect as documented in the medical literature.

Though we can't make the earth as pristine as it once was, we can take proactive steps to minimize our total burden of toxins and ongoing exposures that we will discuss in future chapters.

Supporting Diversity

Each item that passes our lips and travels through our GI tract adds to or subtracts from our overall health savings account. There is a reason that scientists currently believe that upwards of 80 percent of the immune system resides in the GI tract. The 80% number may be true, or it may be a result of not understanding that the MMM exists throughout the body, not just in the GI tract.

Not only do friend and foe microbes enter orally, but so do food allergens, food triggering sensitivities, chemicals, and other pollutants. We must be more selective when we are eating essential nutrients and calories that fuel the trillions of cells that make up our body. These nutrients also fuel the GI microbiota that covers our mucosal membranes and, ultimately, the microbial-mucosal milieu.

Reality is that our microbiome and microbiota diversity is uniquely individual, with no two humans having the same ecosystem and thus MMM. And a person's MMM is constantly adapting throughout the body.

A microbiome with high diversity has the tools in its arsenal to support a healthy milieu anywhere in the body. Just as stem cells are created and stored in bone marrow, the GI tract and appendix are primary repositories of microbial diversity.

Birth and Childhood

Each individual begins to establish their GI tract and whole-body microbiome in the mother's placenta (*in utero*) and continues throughout childhood.[2] Thus when attempting to regain a more robust health status, literally examining a given person's microbial diversity journey is essential.

It has been shown in countless medical journal articles that even your birth order within your family determines your microbial diversity, susceptibility to allergies, and immune competence.[3] In turn, there is clear evidence that a vaginal birth dramatically impacts GI flora, enhancing diversity and volume of the fledgling MMM.[4] Also, a hospital birth vs. home birth may make a difference.[5] Needless to say, any medical interventions and interactions with hospital staff or sterilizing (cleaning) agents can directly alter microbial diversity. After all, nosocomial infections (hospital infections and germs) are well documented. Also, if an infant is breastfed, he or she will be exposed to maternal MMM, such as mother's colostrum, milk, and microbiota on the skin and the breast surface.

Care for the newborn infant, toddler, and child are also factors that can influence microbial diversity. Food prepared by various individuals will bring exposure to their unique microbial profile. In turn, if a child is raised with pets, it can positively impact their microbial diversity and immune competence. [6]

Who's in the Kitchen

In Chapter 9 we will discuss all food factors, not just pathogens. These include dietary diversity, GMO, organic, nutrient depleted foods, irradiated food, homogenized, vegetarian, and the harmful effects of ingested alkalinity.

Indeed, food selection is paramount to creating and sustaining a healthy microbiota and thus is part of establishing a healthy, dynamic MMM. Dietary considerations will be discussed in chapter 9. We will discuss exposure to pathogens that can impact the MMM. Whether it is foodborne illness or exposure to a parasite, amoeba, or similar organism, the root of exposure is contaminated water or food with a common denominator, fecal contamination. It's reasonable to suggest sanitary practices in food handling while trying to rebalance an altered MMM.

Likewise, your exposure to broader dietary diversity could be astronomically higher if you frequently eat out at a variety of ethnic and varied restaurants where food is freshly prepared. Fast food and fast casual dining restaurants will have the opposite effect on your microbial diversity. Ultimately, your health and safety is dependent on the education, attention to detail, and care applied to food preparation, including the rinsing off of fresh produce before prepping. By not rinsing off the food, you have more of a chance of being exposed to dangerous contaminants than you do of exposing yourself to probiotics found in soil.

We each have unique susceptibility as captured in the diagram below. This is merely an example of what happens if there is low stomach acid from aging, medication, or fad pseudoscience, such as alkaline water.

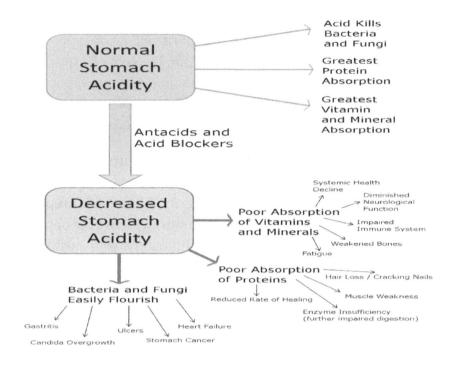

Who's in the Bathroom?

It is self-evident that bathrooms at home or in public are not hygienic. Indeed, it would be the rare person that washes their hands before flushing the toilet. Thus, the toilet handle is contaminated with human microbiota, as is the bathroom stall door, faucets, paper towel dispenser, and the notorious bathroom door handle.

Medicine is aware of the benefits that the microbiome contracted from other people has on GI health as now evidenced by the use of fecal transplants to treat conditions such as infection with the bacteria *Clostridioides difficile*.

We will further explore these hazards and benefits. So too

will we explore the concept of what is sterile? The question of sterility is raised as we establish that you absorb nutrients (especially vitamins) from the bolus or fecal matter in your colon.

Who's in the Bedroom?

Intimate partner exposure is also considered when looking at shifts in microbiota diversity and the MMM. Just as with food, oral contact with surfaces, human or inanimate, will expose you to potentially new and novel bacterial species. Exposure is exposure, whether it be from the kitchen, bathroom, bedroom, family pet, or garden. The skin is well inoculated, which also speaks to the MMM's expansive reach in the body far beyond the GI tract.

The Reality

Our microbial selves play an integral role in who we are. They impact our thinking and overall existence. They equate to the total number of human cells or exceed them.[7]

Our unique maternal and paternal genetics and individual microbiome also can impact our microbiome and MMM.[7]

Transmission of genetics described above and microbiome described below from parent to progeny is an essential start for life. For instance, research has shown that altered microbiota can contribute to obesity. Thus, it is both nature and nurture that dictates our health throughout life. A heavier parent often has heavier children. Is this from genetics, diet, environment, exercise habits, or the influence of all exposures?[8] In Chapter

2 we will discuss food and environment. In Chapter 9 we will discuss diet and lifestyle.

Clinical Considerations Impacting the Microbiome and MMM

Who is working for whom? The microbiome can actually regulate your thoughts, your mood, and your brain health.

> *"The gut microbiota is associated with brain development and function, as well as altered emotional, motor, and cognitive behaviors in animals."* [9]

We mention this to establish a shared appreciation of the many factors that impact the microbiome and MMM. As we discuss specific organ and tissue microbiota in the following chapters, it will become clear that the philosophy and science of the MMM have been established. The research community is doing an excellent job in advancing the science of the impact of the microbiota, microbiome, metagenome, and even the metabolome. The limitation is integrating the MMM concept from a holistic perspective so that you can use it to eliminate your health challenges. The whole of the MMM is greater than the sum of its parts.

How Diet Impacts the Microbiome and Consequently Your Overall Health

"...the microbiome may be more readily reshaped by environmental factors such as dietary exposures and is increasingly recognized to potentially impact human physiology by participating in digestion, the absorption of nutrients, shaping of the mucosal immune response, and the synthesis or modulation of a plethora of potentially bioactive compounds. Thus, diet-induced microbiota alterations may be harnessed in order to induce changes in host physiology, including disease development and progression."[10]

The authors suggest that the food and microcontaminants a person eats may alter the microbiome, which affects appetite, fermentation and availability of nutrients, fat accumulation, which affect health of the body, as well as cognitive behavior.

Just as cells that comprise the body are vulnerable and responsive to total nutritional status, digestive health, and ingested disruptive factors such as allergens and environmental toxins, so is the microbiota throughout the body vulnerable and responsive to these factors. All of these factors also strengthen or weaken the MMM's ability to protect against imbalances that arise from internal and external threats to sustained homeostasis.

A couple of decades ago, we perceived the brain as protected by an essentially impermeable and protective blood-brain barrier (BBB), the ultimate shield of the neurons of our central nervous system. Research has found that the BBB is vulnerable to damage via leaky gut, known as leaky brain.[11] Leaky gut—what scientists call increased intestinal permeability—refers to a weakened gut lining. This allows undigested food particles and pathogenic bacteria to slip through the intestinal walls into systemic circulation, causing problems throughout the body, including the brain.

Now we hypothesize that the entry and exit of nutrients, waste, and contaminants through the BBB are controlled by the MMM, which is an integral part of the BBB. The MMM supports and protects the function of the BBB.

> "The human gut contains trillions of bacterial cells that are reported to be at a ratio of approximately 1:1 with our own cells. Thus, they (the bacteria or MMM) form a vibrant living population that has metabolic activity similar to the liver. There is consequently a move to describe the microbiota, as a whole, a new human organ."[12]

This demonstrates that research scientists are coming close to arriving at a similar, albeit limited, concept of the MMM. Describing the microbiota as an organ is partially true. But the MMM acts more like a system than an organ, such as the vascular, lymph, and ATP systems. The microbiota isn't the only factor that comes into play with cellular and biochemical communication identified by MMM theory. Scientists go on to speak of the integral importance of the intestinal mucosa, a very forward-looking concept. Yet, regarding the MMM, it is vitally important not to limit our look at merely GI microbiota or mucosa.

> "Their [the microbiota's] intimate association with the intestinal mucosa, which is also highly biologically active with a high cellular turnover rate, can be expected to have a major impact on human health and the prevention or precipitation of disease. The gut microbiota has a symbiotic relationship with the host, playing a role in maintaining health and metabolic homeostasis through the production of many metabolites. The collective genomes of these micro-organisms that inhabit the gut are referred to as the metagenome. The development of the gut microbiome begins before birth and in healthy individuals is largely completed within three years, but can be modified by environmental factors, particularly diet composition and volume, and antibiotic therapy."[12]

The lack of maturity of a child's microbiome reflects the heightened level of susceptibility of kids to altered GI, sinus, and all other organ integrity and serves as a source of vulnerability to the entire body's biochemical and physiological processes.

> "Recent studies have suggested that the intestinal microbiome plays an important role in modulating the risk of several chronic diseases, including inflammatory bowel disease, obesity, type 2 diabetes, cardiovascular disease, and cancer. At the same time, it is now understood that diet plays a significant role in shaping the microbiome, with

experiments showing that dietary alterations can induce large, temporary microbial shifts within 24 hours. Given this association, there may be significant therapeutic utility in altering microbial composition through diet."[13]

A composite of the five M's—Microbiota, Microbiome, Metagenome, Metabolome, Mucosal-Terrain—yields the MMM-combined effect that exerts a pervasive influence locally and globally throughout the body. Much like a pebble dropped into a lake, the result reaches far beyond the point of impact. Magnify this effect by trillions of pebbles, each with their competing sphere of influence, and we see the impact to any alteration of the MMM.

Knowing that the skin, organs, and tissues throughout the body each have their microbiome interacting with all other interconnected microbiomes, we must multiply the numbers shared here by many fold. In the GI tract, most microbiotas reside within the more distal parts of the digestive tract, where their biomass surpasses 1,011 cells per gram.[14]

Beyond the presence of select microbes in the gut is their contribution to biosynthesis of vitamins, essential amino acids, and metabolic byproducts from dietary components purposefully unprocessed by the small intestine. Among these byproducts of microbial metabolism are short chain fatty acid (SCFA) byproducts such as butyrate, propionate, and acetate that serve as a primary energy source for cells lining the intestines and may therefore strengthen the mucosal barrier.[13]

Notes For Scientists and Clinicians

Mucosal health is achieved by creating a fertile environment for the microbiota to reside and then delivering nutrients essential for host health, also ensuring self-preservation.

As we proceed through our presentation of MMM Theory, we will examine how the local and total MMM impacts various systems (such as circulatory, energy, nervous, and behavioral) and organs throughout the body. Chapter 9 will explore specific impacts of diet and lifestyle on the microbial-mucosa milieu.

As we explore the role of the MMM throughout the following chapters, we'll discuss the effect of diet, lifestyle, and supplementation and their relationship to alterations in the MMM. For example, a short-term change in diet—such as to one that is strictly animal-based or plant-based—alters microbial composition within just 24 hours of beginning the diet, reversing to baseline within 48 hours of diet discontinuation.[14] Likewise, consider the research on the hormonal disruption and circadian impact seen in the gut microbiome of animals fed a high-fat or high-sugar diet.[14]

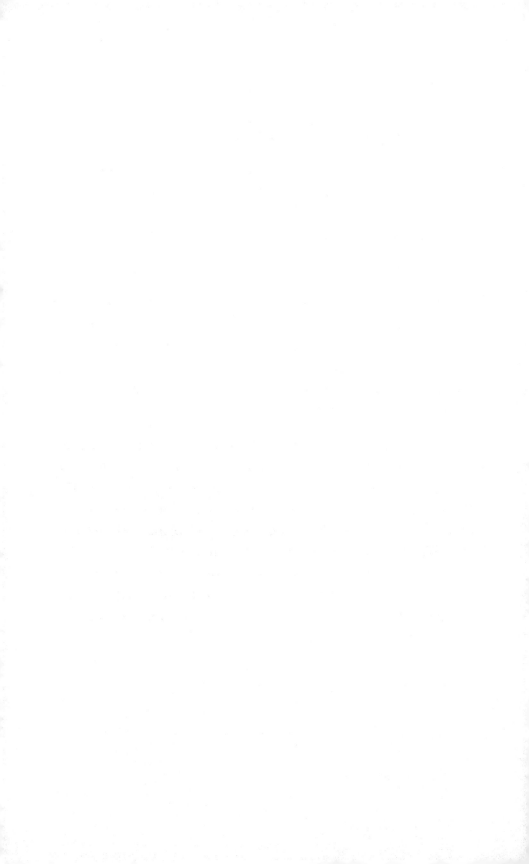

CHAPTER TWO

YOU ARE BEING POISONED!

Are you being poisoned? The answer is a resounding YES. Our food supply is contaminated. The air is contaminated. Your water is contaminated. The soil is contaminated. Many things you use in your home and at work carry poisons. Am I an alarmist? Read on and see if you too are concerned about reaching toxic overload from these man-made chemicals.

If we are all being poisoned, why doesn't everyone know about it? That's what we will reveal in this book, as well as how these unseen and misunderstood microcontaminants are harming you.[1] And what you can do to stay healthy.

Likewise, why isn't everyone sick? We each have a different tipping point—the point where the body burden of contaminants overwhelms our body and its protective mechanisms. This point is where you show distinct symptoms. We all have different strengths and weaknesses in our bodies. Those can emanate from genetic strengths and weaknesses, prior disease or injury, the quality of your diet, the environment where you live and work, and most importantly, the strength and weaknesses of your protective MMM.

Throughout this book, we will tell you how you are being poisoned by things that most people think are harmless. Doctors call the means by which something harms your body "mechanisms of action" and "pathways."

In this chapter, we will help you identify what is poisoning you and causing your body to react. These reactions are often called inflammation, disease, autoimmune disease, or a varying set of symptoms which causes your doctors to send you to several specialists who don't come to the same diagnosis, likely because they are trained to look at the symptoms, rather than for the cause.

I would say that if you have a "disease" that your doctors just can't identify, this chapter and book are especially important to you and your doctors. I use disease in quotation marks because I don't really consider poisoning a disease.

Allopathic medicine and pharmaceutical companies love identifying dysbiosis (the body acting out of harmony or acting up) as a disease. It gives them exclusive rights to diagnose and sell you, and your insurance company remedies. It's extremely profitable. Sometimes the remedy acts as a second poison (prescription drug side effects, mitochondrial damage, stomach upset, skin irritation, and more) to your body as it tries to treat your symptoms.

An admonition I have been using for years when you don't understand why something is occurring is "follow the money."

What is a Poison?

There are two kinds of poison we will discuss. The first kind destroys body tissue and body systems directly. These poisons include acids, hydrocarbons (gasoline, tar, benzene, toluene, parabens, phthalates, etc.) and heavy metals.

The more insidious poisons weaken or disable your body's protective barriers – your microbial mucosal milieu (MMM) – so that other poisons or microcontaminants can enter your body and circulate through the vascular, blood-brain barrier, lymph, glymphatic (a nutrient delivery and waste-clearance system for the central nervous system (CNS)), gastrointestinal, urinary tract, and other pathways. These MMM poisons include herbicides, pesticides, alcohol, chlorine, chloramine, cleaning chemicals, hydrocarbons, sugar, and countless other modern profitable creations.

Some poisons harm both tissue and your microbiome. These include alkaline water and radiation, such as 5G broadcasts.

The Poisons Lurking Among Us

Herbicides

The herbicide most used in the U.S. is glyphosate. Monsanto markets it under the brand name Roundup. It's interesting to find out that Bayer Pharmaceuticals acquired Monsanto in 2018. While one division of Bayer profits from poisoning you, another division profits from providing solutions to your pain, a novel implementation of vertical business integration.

Monsanto has found a new use for Roundup, the most widely used herbicide in the U.S. – as a drying agent that keeps food from spoiling while being transported and in storage. While you can't wash out the glyphosate that is absorbed into your food while it is growing, be sure to wash your fruits and vegetables to at least remove surface herbicides.

Glyphosate

Glyphosate is the active ingredient in Roundup®, a herbicide used to kill weeds growing among crops.

Glyphosate, like other organophosphates, disrupts the shikimate pathway, which governs synthesis of phenylalanine, tyrosine, and tryptophan.

Genetically Modified (GM) crops are designed to withstand large amounts of glyphosate, by use of alternate enzyme pathways. Glyphosate absorbed by plants is concentrated as it passes up the food chain—for example, when corn, soy, hay, and alfalfa are used as feed for cattle, pigs, chickens, and other animals.

The shikimate pathway is found in plants, algae, fungi, bacteria, and other organisms but not in mammals.

Thus, glyphosate does not directly kill humans and animals, it just destroys the MMM.

Destroying the MMM exposes humans and animals to environmental contaminants, which cause inflammatory cascades throughout their bodies.

Glyphosate is toxic to Enterococcus, Bacillus, and Lactobacillus, key components of the human and animal MMM, bacteria which prevent proliferation of Clostridioides difficile (C. diff.), a bacterium that causes diarrhea and inflammation of the colon (colitis).

These disruptions have been connected to digestive issues, obesity, autism, Alzheimer's, depression, Parkinson's, liver diseases, and cancer. [2-4]

Monsanto sells genetically modified corn and soy that are resistant to glyphosate. This means that the Monsanto crops can withstand heavier doses of glyphosate without harming the herbicide-tolerant plants. This is the epitome of GMO fears – a genetically modified organism – corn and soy seeds, that grow as plants that can tolerate and deliver more glyphosate to your dining table.

There is growing evidence that glyphosate could harm the soil and affect the health of the farmers who use it. In addition, studies have shown that consuming glyphosate-containing foods is bad for your health.

Glyphosate is a broad-spectrum herbicide that kills many plants, including crops that are planted in fields. It is targeted for weeds by using it on corn, wheat, and soybean crops. These crops are used in over two hundred products, including food, clothing, household items, toys, and cosmetics.

Glyphosate works by killing the plant's roots, killing the germinating seeds, and killing the shoots that emerge from the seed. It is a broad-spectrum herbicide that affects a wide variety of weeds. However, it has the same effect on beneficial plants. Therefore, Monsanto created special plant seeds whose genes are modified to withstand the herbicide. It happens to be that these seeds do not grow plants that produce their own seeds. So, once a farmer covers their fields in glyphosate, they are compelled to purchase new seeds from Monsanto every season.

Glyphosate is highly water soluble and therefore readily leaches out of the soil and into water supplies.

The U.S. EPA has determined that glyphosate does not pose any health risks to humans based mostly on studies sponsored by and provided to them by Monsanto. More and more studies are showing that glyphosate is likely to cause cancer. In addition, studies have shown that people who eat diets that contain foods that were grown with glyphosate-containing herbicides have higher levels of glyphosate in their urine than those who eat diets that do not contain this herbicide.

Thirty-three countries have banned the use of glyphosate. It is banned in:

- **Argentina**
- **Australia (in some states)**
- **Austria**
- **Bahrain**
- **Barbados**
- **Belgium**
- **Bermuda**
- **Brazil**
- **Canada (8 out of 10 provinces)**
- **Colombia**

- Costa Rica
- Czech Republic
- Denmark
- El Salvador
- Fiji
- France
- Germany
- India
- Italy
- Luxembourg
- Malta
- Netherlands
- Oman
- Portugal
- Qatar
- Saudi Arabia
- Scotland
- Slovenia
- Spain
- Sri Lanka
- St. Vincent and the Grenadines
- Thailand
- Vietnam

But NOT the United States!

If you are buying food items that may be imported, such as wine, beer, beef, lamb, organic fruits and vegetables, look for products from these countries. Based on anecdotal evidence, it is less likely to get a hangover from adult beverages that are produced from plants that are grown without glyphosate! I wonder why.

Alcohol

Generally, there are two types of alcohol – the kind you drink and the antiseptic/antibacterial. Both are harmful to the MMM in the same way. But one of them is much more fun!

Alcohol cleaners are intended to kill bacteria. Like most cleaners, alcohol is non-specific – it kills both good and harmful bacteria. It leaves a bacterial void in its wake. That void is filled by the most available and persistent bacteria in the local environment.

One analogy is a farm. At the end of a growing season, if the farmer plows over and kills all the plants growing on his farm, he has the option of reseeding or leaving the land to grow wild. If he reseeds, he has control over what will grow next. If he leaves it up to chance as to what will grow, it will likely begin as weeds, and continue with the most prevalent local plants, whether they are indigenous or from other farms in the area. Does he want to harvest whatever may grow? No, he wants to maximize his harvest for the best plants in terms of water needed, marketplace needs and value, nutrients needed, herbicides needed, and eventually profitability for his farm.

You want the same control after you consume alcohol. Either you leave it to chance as to which strains of bacteria repopulate your gut and elsewhere in your body, or you "seed" your gut with a diversity of beneficial bacteria, such as in a probiotic formulation or fermented foods.

Wine, beer, sake, and liquor all contain alcohol. There are lots of scientific studies which support most any opinion you have on drinking, such as it is beneficial in moderate doses, or it is harmful. In either case, alcohol acts as an antibacterial, damaging your microbiome and MMM throughout your G.I. tract. Taking a probiotic before drinking reduces the intoxicating effect of alcohol. Taking a probiotic after drinking helps your body repopulate with beneficial bacteria.

As I mentioned above, anecdotal evidence supporting MMM Theory indicates that it is much harder to get a hangover from adult beverages produced from plants grown without glyphosate!

Antibiotics

The purpose of antibiotics is to destroy bacteria.

Antibiotics in general exhibit limited selectivity between the 10% harmful and the 90% beneficial bacteria.

So they may kill the harmful bacteria, but they cause 9x collateral damage and wipe the slate clean so a new mix of harmful and beneficial bacteria can repopulate.

Antibiotics may very well be indicated when bacterial infection is confirmed.

Rather than trying to kill every last harmful bacterium (old model), we suggest introducing probiotics to repopulate and balance remaining harmful bacteria which will always coexist.

Collateral damage of MMM dysbiosis may present as:

- Inflammation, G.I. issues, reoccurring infections, and diseases that are said to be a result of inflammation.
- "Autoimmune disease".
- Organ disease – cardiovascular, pulmonary, kidney, liver, G.I., rheumatic.
- Diseases of development and aging.

The purpose of antibiotics is to destroy bacteria causing an infection or illness. While this is often the best remedy for an infection, most doctors and pharmaceutical companies do not think about the next step in the life cycle of your gut, or the MMM in the rest of your body. It is better to think like a farmer, and "reseed" your intestinal tract and the MMM proliferation throughout your body with beneficial bacteria. Most antibiotic prescriptions are prescribed with directions for use, but leave it to chance as to what bacteria will repopulate your gut and everywhere else.

In addition, many antibiotics are so broad that while they address an infection in the target area, such as the sinuses or lungs, they also affect beneficial bacteria in the gastrointestinal tract, skin, oral microbiome, vagina, and other organs. Thus the microbial mucosal milieu throughout the body becomes disturbed, imbalanced, and susceptible.

Pharmaceutical companies identify the immediate and short-term side effects of the antibiotic in the drug insert. The major side effects are symptoms of a damaged microbiome or MMM in the gastrointestinal tract, such as diarrhea, vomiting, loose stools, and recurring infection. Drug inserts tend to say that the side effects can appear up to a few months after taking the antibiotic. However, antibiotic damage to beneficial bacteria is long term.

Therefore it is critically important to take a probiotic which is resistant to antibiotics, such as sporing probiotics – beneficial probiotics that multiply quickly, such as *Bacillus coagulans* – before, during, and after treatment with antibiotics. In a pinch, and after treatment with antibiotics, almost any probiotic will help the patient recover their decimated G.I. tract back to healthy normal.

Ground-Breaking Antibiotic Research

As I write this, I see a new research report where scientists have created a trojan horse procedure to encapsulate antibiotics within red blood cells (RBC) for targeted delivery of high-potency and highly toxic antibiotics to specific harmful bacteria.

The trojan horse RBC, described in a September 2022 paper in the journal ACS Infectious Diseases, could help to address the worsening antibiotic resistance, say the scientists.[5] These scientists are physicists, not biologists or physicians, at McMaster University, Ontario, Canada. They also modified and tested red blood cells as a carrier for one of the world's only remaining highly resistant antibiotics Polymyxin B (PmB), often considered a treatment of last resort due to its toxic and dangerous side effects, which include kidney damage.

PmB is used to fight particularly dangerous and frequently medicine-resistant bacteria similar to E. coli, which is responsible for many serious conditions such as pneumonia, gastroenteritis, and bloodstream infections.

These physicists developed a way to open red blood cells and remove the inner factors, leaving only a membrane — known as a liposome, which can be loaded with medicine molecules and inserted back into the body.

The process also involves sheathing the outside of the red blood cell membrane with antibodies, allowing it to stick to target bacteria and deliver the drug safely.

This trojan horse RBC delivery system may prevent much of the collateral damage done by antibiotics. I wonder if there are any implications for the blood or blood brain barrier MMM.

Chlorine and Chloramines

Tap water is a source of chlorine and chloramines that are used in urban water supplies to keep bacteria from growing in the water delivery system.[6,7] That is great, but chlorine remains in the water when you drink it, shower, and bathe with it. It kills your protective MMM (beneficial bacteria which protects your body from other environmental contaminants).

In addition to the harmful effect chloramines have on your MMM, the newer chloramines have a disastrous effect on copper pipes over time. They soften the copper so that after a few years, new copper plumbing will start springing pinhole leaks inside your walls. These pinhole leaks are usually not caught immediately, but when they are found, they are often accompanied with mold growth in your walls and on porous wallboard. Those chloramines which save your water company

a few pennies per thousand gallons, may end up costing you thousands of dollars in repairs many times.

Copper pipe was installed in houses, either before public water companies started using chloramines or after plumbers learned from experience that copper pipes spring pinhole leaks in certain neighborhoods. Water pipe is generally never installed so it is accessible without ripping out walls, ceilings, floors, and more. Your plumber and general contractor should know better by now.

Some plumbers and contractors will try to upgrade you to heavier duty copper pipes to reduce the chances of pinhole leaks in your walls. Thicker and more expensive copper pipes will last longer before they spring leaks. The best way I know to use copper pipes is to use a whole house chlorine and chloramine water filter. Be sure to ask if the water filter you are considering removes chloramines as well as chlorine, as it is chloramines which soften copper.

I learned the hard way to also ask about maintenance of your whole house water filter. When I first moved into my new house, I heard this loud flow of water. It turns out that the water filter was backflushing to clean its filters. It backflushes for 20 minutes twice per month. In Los Angeles, this uses about $80 of water to clean the water filter monthly. Not only is it costly, but it is such a waste of water, flowing full force through the water filter into the sewage system. Where water is precious, such as in Los Angeles, which is essentially a desert climate, it is such a disservice that people who sell water filters don't mention that this water waste occurs regularly. I can cut my water usage and plant indigenous plants that use little water, but then have to listen to water flowing full force through my water filter into the sewer.

An alternative to copper is PEX plastic pipe. PEX is supposed to be safe for both hot and cold water. I wonder if we will learn the same about PEX that we learned about plastic water bottles, Teflon, and other products long after use began. While you can replace a plastic water bottle or Teflon pan with safer materials, you are basically stuck with the choice of piping in your home.

Cleaning chemicals

Cleaning agents/chemicals can stay on one's clothes, dishes, household and office surfaces, all contributing to the disruption of the MMM[8] quietly working in the background to ensure you are exposed to MMM damaging chemicals for a long time.

Acetaminophen

Researchers report that acetaminophen use has been linked to the marked increase in autism spectrum disorder (ASD), asthma, and ADHD.

As well, environmental contaminants – pesticides, chemicals, phthalates, polychlorinated biphenyls, solvents, heavy metals, or other pollutants - are linked to ASD.

Acetaminophen causes severe immune abnormalities at doses that do not damage the liver.

As of Oct 2013, 2,685 articles indexed in PubMed discuss acetaminophen toxicity.

As of 2012, 145 studies have shown a link between mitochondrial function and autism.[9]

Hypothesis: acetaminophen damages the MMM contributing to immune reaction, mitochondrial dysfunction, autism, asthma, ADHD, dementia, and Alzheimer's.

Habitual use of acetaminophen greater than 2,000 milligrams per day has been associated with a 3.7 times increased threat of bleeding in the upper gastrointestinal tract.[10] Acetaminophen can also cause intestinal permeability. Overdose with acetaminophen causes necrosis of liver tissue, which releases a protein that results in leakage of harmful bacteria from the gut into the bloodstream.[11]

Heavy Metals

Heavy metals are naturally occurring pollutants and may include arsenic, cadmium, lead, mercury, and nickel. They have been associated with several adverse health effects, such as immune system suppression, hormonal dysregulation and gut dysbiosis. Heavy metals in the gut are also associated with increased inflammation, oxidative stress, and metabolic dysfunction.

While fluoride in public water systems and toothpaste is not a metal, fluoride additives contain heavy metal toxins that must be diluted to meet drinking water regulations. Heavy metal content varies by batch, and in one study all samples contained arsenic (4.9–56.0 ppm) or arsenic in addition to lead (10.3 ppm).[12] Some samples contained barium (13.3–18.0 ppm) instead. All fluoride samples contained a surprising amount of aluminum—thus the warning on commercial toothpaste not to swallow the pleasantly flavored toothpaste. If more than a small amount is swallowed, "get medical

help or contact a Poison Control Center right away." This is especially difficult with kids, but the package says to "supervise children's brushing and rinsing to avoid swallowing." That's easy.

Several strains of *Lactobacillus* have demonstrated the capacity to effectively bind to and sequester heavy metals from water in animal cell models.[13-15]

Studies suggest that enhancing microbial conditions in the gut microbiome with probiotics helps to prevent heavy metal absorption, translocation, and permeability in the intestines.[13,14,16,17] Still, the impact of heavy metal toxins extends beyond the gut and impacts other organ systems such as the kidneys, liver, and brain.[18-20]

Probiotics may enhance enzyme production and their effectiveness in detoxification, with some studies suggesting that the beneficial bacteria's modulatory effect on bile acid production is one way that may support the healthy excretion of heavy metals.[13,16,17,21]

Lactobacillus casei and Lactobacillus plantarum are called out in the studies supporting increased bile glutathione production and fecal bile acid excretion.[13,16,17,21] These studies give preliminary substantiation for the roll of probiotics in supporting enterohepatic circulation, the movement of bile acid molecules from the liver to the small intestine and back to the liver. [13,16,17,21]

Toxic Chemicals

Ultimately our body's elaborate and sophisticated detoxification systems become overloaded, which leads to the emergence of acute and chronic conditions – conditions that conventional medicine frequently diagnose as some kind of disease. Environmental toxicity is not well established as a cause of disease, especially its effect on the MMM. Thus these "diseases" are treated by suppressing symptoms of the body's response to poisoning with patented drugs and pharmaceutical biologics.

Please read chapter 9: Diet, Lifestyle, and Supplement Considerations for ways to detoxify your body of these toxic chemicals.

- Perchlorate toxicity – perchlorate is a component in jet fuel and fireworks that extensively contaminates the air and our food. It's now found in disturbing amounts in breast milk and urine. Perchlorate is a well-known endocrine disrupter with the ability to block iodine receptors in the thyroid, contributing to hypothyroidism and attendant neurological dysfunction.[22]

- Pesticide toxicity – Lactic acid bacterial strains isolated from kimchi, the Korean fermented cabbage dish, have been shown to degrade four different organophosphorus insecticides. These lactic acid strains use organophosphorus insecticides as a source of carbon and phosphorus.[23,24]

- Bisphenol-A (BPA) toxicity – Bisphenol A has become a ubiquitous toxicant derived from petrochemicals. BPA has endocrine-disrupting properties. It has been shown to accumulate in the food chain, at the top of which are humans. BPA has been linked to a wide range of health problems. Certain probiotic strains have been demonstrated in animal models to both reduce the intestinal absorption of BPA and enhance its excretion.[25]

- Gluten toxicity – Wheat and gluten have increasingly been linked as a contributing factor in a wide range of health problems, with up to 300 potential adverse effects identified. Certain probiotic strains may reduce the immunotoxic properties of gluten peptides by degrading them into non-toxic peptides.[26] Interestingly, the mouth has lately been found to contain bacteria capable of degrading gluten, indicating there may be other gluten-degrading microorganisms within the upper gastrointestinal tract. Something as simple as what your mother told you such as to completely chew your food may reduce the potential antigenicity/immunotoxicity of wheat gluten peptides.[27]

- Aspirin toxicity – Pharmaceutical companies and some doctors recommend drugs such as aspirin for its preventive role in heart disease, despite the fact that even low dose aspirin use causes intestinal injury and other serious adverse health effects. Though aspirin's adverse health effects have been established in the literature to far outweigh its purported health benefits, millions take it on a daily basis without full knowledge of how it's affecting them. Certain probiotic strains have been shown to reduce the MMM and gastrointestinal damage done by aspirin.[28] There are much better means to keep your blood flowing, such as Japanese fermented cheese natto and supplements containing nattokinase.

Ralph Holsworth, D.O. has done extensive research and written about nattokinase as a safer alternative to low dose aspirin. "Nattokinase is a particularly potent treatment because it enhances the body's natural ability to fight blood clots in several different ways and has many benefits including convenience of oral administration, confirmed efficacy, prolonged effects, cost effectiveness, and can be used preventatively. It is a naturally occurring, food dietary supplement that has demonstrated stability in the gastrointestinal tract. The properties of nattokinase closely resemble those properties of plasmin so it dissolves fibrin directly! More importantly, it also enhances the body's production of both plasmin and other clot dissolving agents, including urokinase. Nattokinase may actually be superior to conventional clot-dissolving drugs such as urokinase, and streptokinase, which are only effective therapeutically when taken intravenously within 12 hours of a stroke or heart attack. Nattokinase, however, may help prevent the conditions leading to blood clots with an oral daily dose of as little as 2,000 fibrin units (F.U.)." from *Blood Circulation Nattokinase*, by Dr. Holsworth.[29]

- Sodium Nitrate toxicity – numerous foods are preserved with nitrates, which may form DNA-damaging nitrosamines. Kimchi derived Lactic acid bacteria have been shown to degrade sodium nitrate.[30]

- Vaccine toxicity – there is a lot of controversial literature describing the unintended adverse side effects of vaccines. These side effects frequently far exceed the vaccines purported benefits. These studies are not sponsored by the pharmaceutical companies which market the vaccines. This is especially true for attenuated live vaccines, such as oral polio vaccine, which have lately been linked to thousands of cases of childhood vaccine induced paralysis in countries like India. A beneficial form of yeast has been shown in a recent animal study to prevent oral polio vaccine-induced IgA nephropathy, a form of immune-mediated kidney damage.[31] Also, probiotic bacteria have been shown to positively regulate the two poles of immunity (TH1/ TH2), which vaccines frequently upset by inducing hypersensitization via over-activation of the adaptive/humoral (TH2) pole of immunity.[32]

- Chemotherapy toxicity – No chemical therapy is more fraught with life-changing risks than chemotherapy – used to treat already very sick and weak patients. Some chemotherapy agents, such as the nitrogen mustard class, are so poisonous that they bear chemical munitions designations, and are banned by the Chemical Weapons Convention. There's evidence that a specific probiotic is able to reduce the adverse effects on immune health induced by chemotherapy agents.[33]

Sugar

Sugar is an indirect MMM poison. While it does not directly harm the MMM, it promotes growth of harmful bacteria, which causes the microbiome to become unbalanced and unhealthy.

Artificial Sweeteners and Maltodextrin

Artificial sweeteners such as sucralose (Splenda) and aspartame (Equal) promote the growth and adherence of E. coli bacteria.

Researchers at the Cleveland Clinic identify that artificial sweeteners sucralose and aspartame both contain maltodextrin, a common food additive. It is possible that the maltodextrin component of the artificial sweeteners is the culprit, for the natural sweetener Stevia did not have the same E. Coli- Promoting effect.

The Cleveland Clinic researchers repeated their analysis with just maltodextrin and found the same E. Coli-promoting effect. Watch out for maltodextrin, which is in so many processed foods.

On its own, maltodextrin can spike blood sugar, so it is problematic for people with diabetes or reactive hypoglycemia. This is due to its high glycemic index of 106-136, which means that it promotes the rapid release of glucose, thus raising one's blood sugar.

Food processors add maltodextrin to many foods, some of which are assumed to be healthy, such as:

- Weight-training supplements
- Yogurt
- Nutrition bars
- Sauces
- Spice mixes
- Baked goods

- Beer
- Cereals
- Chips
- Artificial sweeteners
- Snack foods
- Candies
- Soft drinks, and others

Are all these foods recognized as highly processed and to be avoided by someone trying to stay healthy?

The FDA lists maltodextrin among generally recognized as safe (GRAS) food additives.

How is maltodextrin made? Maltodextrin is a type of highly processed carbohydrate. It is a white powder processed from rice, corn, wheat, or potato starch. First it's cooked, then acids or enzymes are added to process it some more. The final stage of maltodextrin is a water-soluble white powder with a neutral taste. Maltodextrin is used as an additive in the processed foods above to replace sugar and improve their texture, shelf life, and taste.

If you have gluten sensitivity, be careful about eating foods with maltodextrin. The powder has traces of gluten if its source is wheat and you will have a very difficult time finding its source, which may vary in each processed food – seasonally or for any other sourcing or supply chain reason.

Stomach Acid

Stomach acid is a combination of potassium chloride, sodium chloride, and hydrochloric acid.

Combined with digestive enzymes, stomach acids dissolve organic matter – proteins, fat, and carbs.

G.I. epithelial tissue consists of proteins and fat.

Without a healthy mucosal milieu, these chemicals will digest the surface tissue lining the G.I. tract. Below is a picture of a healthy intestinal MMM.

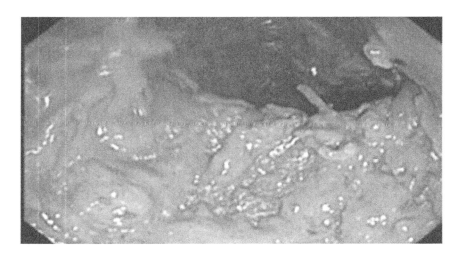

Photo source: mesotheliomacancer1.info

You have likely seen pictures of someone who has spilled acid on their skin. The MMM of the skin is not adapted to protect against strong acids. If it was similar to the MMM in your gut, your skin would look like a monster in a bad movie. Your skin might look like the MMM in your G.I. tract.

Mucosal milieu dysbiosis allows damage to the intestinal wall and a subsequent inflammatory cascade causing G.I. distress, which is diagnosed as "disease."

Alkaline Water

What's the worst thing you can drink (among drinks that are supposed to be ok or good for you)?

The answer: Alkaline water!

The Science

A healthy body maintains a cellular and blood plasma pH in a very narrow range of 7.35 to 7.45, which is slightly basic or alkaline. Basic and alkaline mean the same thing and may be used interchangeably.

On the pH scale, strongly acidic is 0 and strongly alkaline is 14. A pH of 7 is neutral. The pH scale is logarithmic. This means that a pH of 3 is 10 times as acidic as a pH of 4 and 100 times as acidic as a pH of 5.

The stomach maintains a highly acidic pH of 1.5 to 3.5. This acid level helps the stomach digest food and is the proper environment for digestive enzymes to function. Acidity and digestive enzymes break down proteins into their amino acid components. They also help kill harmful bacteria, viruses, mold, mycotoxins, and other living microcontaminants.

Health problems can knock blood pH balance off its normal slightly alkaline range. When your blood pH drops below 7.35, it is referred to as acidosis and when blood becomes more alkaline it is called alkalosis. The kidneys and lungs help to maintain blood pH in its normal range. Kidneys remove acids through urine and the lungs remove carbon dioxide by exhaling it.

Foods that metabolize to enhance blood alkalinity tend to be fruits and vegetables, which can even be acidic when eaten, but are digested and metabolized and end up in the bloodstream as slightly alkaline.

The Pseudo-Science

Some marketeers propose that if you eat and drink alkaline food and liquids, they will increase your blood plasma pH to a higher and more healthy alkaline level. Without diving into biochemistry, this could make sense.

However, often the opposite is true. And balance is the body's goal, not an extreme level of blood alkalinity.

The Effects of Alkaline Water

Quenching your thirst with artificially enhanced alkaline water has the immediate effect of neutralizing your stomach acid.

Without the benefit of stomach acid, lots of bad things happen. Your food is not properly digested, so you do not free the amino acids from proteins and do not release many other micronutrients in your food for fermentation and absorption in your intestines. You become undernourished and are lacking in critical nutrients which may have been in your food.

Furthermore, a lack of stomach acid and acid-thriving digestive enzymes results in intestinal fermentation of carbs, protein putrefaction, oil and fat rancidity, all contributing to cellular acidity. If you're not digesting your food properly, how much does it matter if you are eating a diet of fast food and fruit loops or a healthy diet?

Professor Bruce Ames, one of my mentors, in his Triage Theory of Aging, demonstrates that the body uses a triage process to allocate scarce micronutrients for critical body functions such as to maintain beating of the heart, lung function and the nervous system, including brain function. The results of episodic or long-term micronutrient scarcity, whether caused by lack of nutrients in your diet or malabsorption (due to drinking alkaline water or otherwise), are that these nutrients are not available for long-term functions such as healthy DNA and RNA replication. Early onset of diseases of aging such as cardiovascular, liver, kidney and brain issues and cancer are the initially undiagnosable, consequential result of nutrient deficiency, no matter the cause.

More obvious signs of micronutrient deficiency include brain fog, low energy levels, lack of stamina, and difficulty fighting off illness. Few doctors would look for undernourishment or malnutrition in a patient who says they eat a healthy diet. And few patients would mention that they are poisoning themselves with alkaline water.

The impact of buffered stomach acid includes susceptibility to environmental contaminants entering your body such as harmful bacteria, viruses, mold, and mycotoxins. It does not matter if these pathogens enter your body through breathing or eating. They all end up in your stomach to be killed.

It's obvious that food borne contaminants go to the stomach. It is not so obvious that air borne pathogens also go to the stomach to be killed. However, the function is rather straightforward. Pathogens that you inhale are caught in your lungs. Mucus in the lungs flush the pathogens into your stomach. It's that simple. However, if your stomach acid has been neutralized with alkaline water, these pathogens do not die as they would in a normal highly acidic stomach. They are passed live into your intestines where they may propagate and be absorbed into your body and circulated via the vascular and lymph systems to all your organs. If a patient has a genetic weakness or injury, this is likely where dysfunction or disease will begin to present.

For confirmation, you can look up the side effects of antacids such as omeprazole or Prilosec – Proton Pump Inhibitor (PPI) drugs. Drinking alkaline water has a similar effect to these acid-blocking drugs. And you could experience a pleasant feeling in your stomach temporarily while drinking alkaline water.

People who neutralize their stomach acid whether with drugs or alkaline water have higher counts of *Enterococcus*, *Streptococcus*, *Staphylococcus*, and some strains of *E. Coli*, as well as lower protein/amino acid, and micronutrient absorption.

And alkaline water or PPIs neutralize your body's primary defenses against mold, mycotoxins, harmful bacteria, and viruses. All of these damage your MMM.

This is why I believe that alkaline water is the worst form of hydration you can use.

Effect on Pharmaceutical Drugs

Because most pharmaceutical drugs are formulated and manufactured for oral absorption, neutralizing your stomach acids may enhance, decrease, or have no effect on the absorption of various pharmaceutical drugs.

It's likely that neither your doctor nor pharmacist will be familiar with the effect of neutralizing stomach acid on each drug. It's likely even pharmaceutical researchers have not done studies on this variable, so it is likely you are one of the many alkaline water drinkers who are experimenting on yourself regarding the desired effect and side effects of your medication if you are altering your oral drug absorption pathway.

If you are taking more than one pharmaceutical drug, no one will know what to expect from that combination in an unstudied environment of neutralized stomach acid.

Effect on Herbal Treatments

Herbal treatments have a long history of use in Ayurvedic medicine in places like India, China, and among indigenous people throughout the world.

It is known that some herbs, such as curcumin from turmeric, are difficult to absorb.

Naturopathic doctors, Chinese medicine practitioners, Ayurvedic medicine practitioners, and herbalists likely have little knowledge of the effect of these medicines when stomach acid has been neutralized and the medicines are not broken down in the stomach as has historically occurred. So, in the world of natural medicine, there is likely little understanding of taking medicinal herbs and mushrooms when stomach acids have been neutralized.

Radiation

In the 1950s and 1960s there was fear of radioactive fallout from some tragic event of the Cold War. Monthly, students used to do a drop and cover drill when the school alarm bells were activated. Don't know how that would help with radioactive discharge, but maybe it was a little safer if a conventional missile landed nearby.

Today, electronic radiation is everywhere. Sources of radiation are everywhere – in the home, at work, in a car, in highly electronic buildings, and even if you go camping in the woods and take your cell phone.

Bacteria are very sensitive to radiation. As a matter of fact, radiation is used to kill bacteria in some food distribution processes. Unlike chlorine in your water supply, radiation dissipates after it is used. However, it leaves a barren bacterial field which is open to reestablishment with harmful bacteria, rather than a balance of beneficial and harmful bacteria. There is no bacterial reseeding process after use of radiation on food.

Though highly controversial (follow the money), I believe that electronic broadcasts (radiation) are harmful to your MMM.

There are two sets of data you can explore regarding 5G radiation. Industry sponsored websites such as CTIA Wireless Health Facts, provide evidence and conclude that 5G radiation is safe, given certain guidelines, such as limited exposure. I assume this would apply to someone who doesn't have a cell phone.

I like the information that was submitted to Parliament, U.K. recently.[34] It summarized that human radiation exposure has been increasing exponentially with the use of 3G, then 4G, and now 5G systems.

The authors write: "5G radiation has been shown to induce adverse health effects on living organisms. Studies have revealed it to: inhibit cell proliferation, alter the structure of multiple bodily systems i.e. blood, bone marrow, internal organs, inhibit oxygen uptake in cellular mitochondria, and de-oxygenate your body and lead to respiratory problems, all cellular EMF's are KNOWN to be carcinogens, they damage the structure of DNA, and can induce neurodegeneration i.e. Alzheimer's, all EMF's can result in neurobehavioral dysfunctions like autism, lead to infertility and many, many more issues which will be greatly exacerbated by the progression onto 5G (a more potent frequency)."

On the effects of 5G radiation on bacteria (Soghomonyan et al., 2016) states: "Bacteria and other cells might communicate with each other by electromagnetic field of subextremely high frequency range. This millimeter wavelength (MMW) radiation affects *Escherichia* coli and many other bacteria, mainly depressing their growth and changing properties and activity. These effects were non-thermal and depended on different factors. The significant cellular targets for MMW effects could be water, cell plasma membrane, and genome .... The consequences of MMW interaction with bacteria are the changes in their sensitivity to different biologically active chemicals, including antibiotics .... These effects are of significance for understanding changed metabolic pathways and distinguish role of bacteria in environment; they might be leading to antibiotic resistance in bacteria."

The presentation concludes: "The studies positing the harmful effects of [electromagnetic field] EMF-RF radiation on both human and animal life are endless, though not exhaustive, and undeniably more independent research must be conducted before any concrete conclusions can be reached regarding the physical and ethical boundaries of the use of wireless technology. What is a certainty though, is that at the very least a moratorium should be placed on the roll out of 5G technology in order to address the vast expanse of evidence in the literature which demonstrate the contraindications to the health of humans and the wider ecosystem, which is exuded from the previous generations of EMF's, contraindications which could be greatly exacerbated with the step up to 5G. The people should decide whether to permit technologies which have, over the course of decades, been shown to induce harmful bio-effects and such a decision should not be imposed upon them by governments nor telecommunications companies."

Your Food

Let's start with the easiest discussion.

Toxins in food include herbicides, pesticides, gluten for many people, and GMO food that has been enhanced to withstand (and absorb) a higher dose of herbicides.

We include wine, beer, and spirits in this food category since they are made from fruit, grain, and vegetables. As a rule, I would always choose a wine or beer produced outside the U.S. as having less likelihood of containing pesticides and their residue. You will be surprised how drinking European and Australian wines reduces the likelihood of any hangover symptoms.

Certified organic food is grown without the use of synthetic and chemical herbicides and pesticides. Those chemicals include glyphosate, which is the active ingredient in Roundup. This chemical causes cancer and birth defects in animals and is known to cause damage to humans as well.

Water

Unfortunately, water is a source of toxin exposure in a number of ways including pesticide runoff from farms, excrement runoff from ranches, toxic dumping from factories, acting as a collector of airborne toxins that settle out of the atmosphere, pharmaceutical drugs dumped down the toilet, and many other routes of exposure for many different toxins. Urban water treatment systems were designed to remove sediment, bacteria, and many other contaminants, but not prescription drug molecules created in the laboratory or trace metals, such as aluminum dust which is used to seed rain clouds in farming communities.

Water is a source of chlorine and chloramines that are used in urban water supplies to keep bacteria from growing in the water delivery system. That is great, but chlorine remains in the water when you drink it or shower and bathe with it. It kills your protective microbiome (beneficial bacteria which protect your body from other environmental contaminants).

Water bottled in plastic is often a source of BPA and other unsafe chemicals from plastics, which may act as endocrine disruptors.

Water Filters and Containers

As I mentioned earlier in this chapter, my recommendation: Don't ever drink alkaline water.

Drink the cleanest water you can, on a regular basis. Tap water and standard bottled water have a pH ranging from 6.5 to 7.5. This is fine and healthy.

I choose to use a Reverse Osmosis (R.O.) water filter for my water. The one at the house is a name brand 4-stage under counter filter system. When you shop for an R.O. system, try to find one that has fluoride filtration. But avoid the new technology added to R.O. water filters which alkalinize the water.

One drawback to R.O. filters is that they filter so completely that they remove natural minerals in water. This is where a healthy diet and sophisticated multivitamin/multimineral (with trace minerals) or ionic minerals can supplement your mineral intake.

I carry the R.O. water in a variety of containers, depending on the situation. When I go out to the beach to play volleyball for a few hours I take an insulated stainless-steel canister and include ice from my R.O. supplied icemaker. In my car, I keep a few small, refillable glass bottles that fit in a cup holder. When hiking I use a silicone collapsible water bottle. Occasionally I will use a plastic water bottle for convenience or so I can leave it behind for recycling.

Drink lots of clean, pure water, but don't ever drink alkaline water!

Air

The air we breathe contains environmental contaminants from hydrocarbons, ozone, particulates, smoke, soot, ash, plastics, and depending where you live might also include aluminum dust from rain-inducing efforts, windblown pesticides, herbicides, rubber (from tires on the highway), and many more toxic elements.

Who chooses to live near or downwind of a highway, airport, chemical plant, oil field, refinery, or factory? Well, I have lived near many of them in great neighborhoods in Los Angeles. These neighborhoods included West Hollywood, near the Beverly Center and Cedars Sinai Medical Center, where oil production still takes place, though it is now camouflaged and out of sight. I lived in Beverly Hills, where up until a few years ago, there were working and leaking oil rigs on the high school athletic field adjacent to Century City. I worked in the city of El Segundo in office buildings for 16 years. The city is surrounded by the Hyperion Water Treatment Plant and Chevron Oil Refinery to the west, Los Angeles International Airport (LAX) to the north, and the 405 (one of the busiest highways in the nation) to the east.

We used to watch flare offs at the Chevron Refinery that would sometimes shoot at least 50 feet high. Another time there was an explosion and chemical release where Chevron tried to have everyone in the area have their car detailed so that the chemicals would not remain on the cars and destroy the paint. I asked if there was any concern with inhaling these chemicals that dissolve paint and was told no – don't worry about it.

Then there is the notorious smog in L.A. The horizon used to look greenish brown on bad smog days. It doesn't happen as often due to an immense volume of regulations and investments in California to enhance the cleanliness and safety of the air.

Lately we have had massive fires in California. Not only do these blow ash into the air, they fill the air with burned environmental contaminants that were relatively benign, having settled on the ground. Smoke from the recent California fires has been traced as far away as Europe and even Russia.

Chances are your community has some of these sources of air pollution or others. They damage your MMM and enter your body.

Indoor Environmental Contaminants

Then we head indoors at home, at the office, at the mall, in the car or elsewhere, where the air (and EMF exposure) might be worse. We have off-gassing from plastics, such as a new-car smell. We have high or low VOC (volatile organic compound) paint and varnish residues, carpet off-gassing, pressed wood used in furniture and cabinetry or plywood (glue) off-gassing, and so many other sources of indoor environmental pollution such as mold and mildew that is not cleared by open windows or heating and air conditioning systems.

A lower cost HVAC system is designed to use filters that barely catch large dust particles in the air, let alone small particles such as bacteria, viruses, hydrocarbons, etc. In these systems, you can't just install a higher efficiency filter because it will put too large a drag on the system mechanicals, prematurely wearing out the major units. But you can upgrade the filters to a limited extent without damaging the equipment.

Your lungs are a great filtration system, until they too reach their limit, tipping point, or body burden. What does the body do with the environmental contaminants that it removes from the air? The mucosal system washes those contaminants out of the lungs and deposits them into the gastrointestinal tract (gut), where in susceptible people, that may be the place where air pollution causes the most harm. Who would have thought that air pollution directly affects your G.I. tract?[35]

A contractor story: The painting and general contractors left behind open and partially sealed cans of left-over paint, stacked right next to the heating and air conditioning system and blowers in the garage. This is how to keep your house circulating fresh environmental contaminants for years.

Speaking of the garage, especially if it is attached to the house, there should be an exhaust vent, especially if you use it for cars, not just storage. Your car puts out the most hydrocarbons when starting cold and for hours after being driven.

Cleaning Supplies and "Air Fresheners"

Look at all the warnings on your cleaning supplies – use in a well-ventilated space, avoid prolonged exposure to odor or skin, do not allow to touch skin, rinse for 10 minutes under running water, call a poison control center if … . That's an innocuous way of saying these products are dangerous for humans. I've had contractors totally avoid reading the instructions and warnings. They use chemicals and leave behind a Linus-like cloud of environmental toxins.

I do not recommend any air fresheners. Packaged air fresheners available at the grocery store, pharmacy, or big box stores usually contain hydrocarbon-based esters which smell great, generally not artificial, but damage the MMM in your sinuses, nasal passages, and lungs.

If a remedy is needed, cleaning the source of the smell, mold, mildew, pet dander, cigarette smoke, etc. with non-toxic cleaners, such as mild soap and water, and airing out the space is preferred. Perfuming the pig, especially with hydrocarbon-based chemicals, is not the answer.

Anti-toxin Strategies

Mastering your body and its environment includes:

- Avoid toxins in food, water, and the products you use
- Support your MMM and your gut
- Assist your body to release the toxins
- Repair some of the damage toxins have caused

Fortunately, our bodies have a tremendous capacity for healing and recovery. Take these steps to improve your health now and in the future.

Please see Chapter 9 for more discussion of anti-toxin strategies and supplement recommendations.

CHAPTER THREE

WHERE IS MY MMM?

The graphic on the next page shows the location of your MMM. It is not what anyone would expect.

Your MMM is everywhere in and around your body.

I envisioned and mapped the MMM in a presentation I prepared in 2014, years before research demonstrated plausibility of my MMM Theory and now proves much of it. You will note that most of these studies were published in 2019 – 2022.

It is in your gastrointestinal tract (GIT). This includes your mouth, esophagus, stomach, small and large intestines, appendix, and anus. This is what most people "know."

It is in your sinuses, throat, and lungs.

It is on and in your skin.

It is in every organ in your body – your heart, liver, kidneys, pancreas, and apparently all organs.

It is in every cell in your body.

It is every mitochondrion in your body.

When doctors refer to crosstalk and pathways, they may very well be referring to the way bacteria communicate with their community and communication between bacteria and your body, even though the doctors don't understand the methods or sophistication of these communications. They see that something is happening and put it in the only paradigm that they know.

Your microbiome circulates throughout your body. It presents with different characteristics based on where in the body it exists. Thus, the species, community characteristics, and function of the microbiome differs in different parts of the body.

Your microbiome circulates via several pathways. These include the circulatory systems which we are most familiar with. They include the gastrointestinal tract, the vascular (blood) system, the lymph system, the glymphatic system which delivers nutrients and removes waste from the central nervous system while you are asleep, via movement through interstitial space (the space between cells), and likely more pathways yet to be imagined.

Dr. Meletis coined the term "mmm" to represent localized MMM.

Where is the MMM?

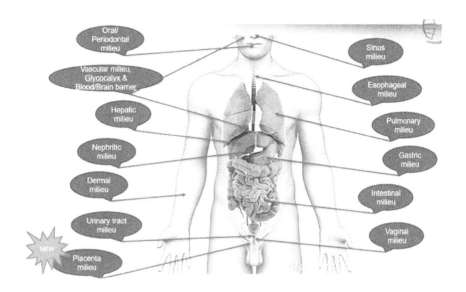

MMM Diversity and Richness

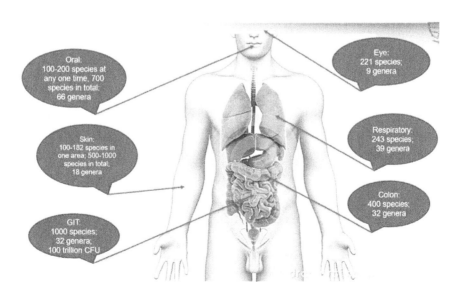

In her 2011 extremely inciteful and novel graduate thesis at Dalhousie University, Halifax, Nova Scotia, STRUCTURE AND FUNCTION OF THE HUMAN MICROBIOME, Marina Lorna Ritchie provides some very provocative information. She has gathered dynamics of the diversity of the microbiome in various organs.

Ritchie identifies network topology of bacterial colonies, ways to define robustness, pattern similarity and differences between the microbiome of different organs, and various ways to measure the results of treatment with probiotics.

In her conclusion, Ritchie identifies food webs that have major implications for human health. She highlights the diverse and complex microbial community as it differs in structure regionally and by age. She recommends a network perspective (rather than a species perspective) to understand microbial communities, their regional impact and perturbations that may one day be used to improve human health.

Pancreatic Microbiome

In a 2019 article published in *Nature Reviews*, doctors Ryan Thomas and Christian Jobin discuss evidence of an inherent pancreatic microbiota as well as the influence of the intestinal microbiota as it relates to pancreatic disease and development.[1] **They discuss microbiota impact on diseases intrinsic to the pancreas such as pancreatitis, pancreatic cancer (pancreatic ductal adenocarcinoma or PDAC), and type 1 diabetes mellitus.**

The article is titled: *Microbiota in pancreatic health and disease: the next frontier in microbiome research.* In the article, the authors examine literature implicating microorganisms in diseases of the pancreas.

In another study titled, *The microbiota and microbiome in pancreatic cancer: more influential than expected*, doctors from the Department of Pancreatic Surgery, Fudan University Shanghai Cancer Center, discuss their findings.[2] This study was published in 2019 in the journal *Molecular Cancer*.

The authors explain that the pancreas was traditionally considered a sterile organ, and it has long been held that most microbes cannot survive in pancreatic juice, which contains numerous proteases and is highly alkaline. Yet, compared with normal pancreatic tissue, a 1,000-fold increase of bacteria in intrapancreatic space was identified in PDAC patients using 16S rRNA florescent probes and qPCR testing.

However, they went further to identify specific microbiota differences in multiple organs of patients with and without PDAC (cancer). They noted differences in oral, GI, and pancreatic tissues.

The study authors note a difference in gut flora and pancreatic flora, and a further difference between patients with and without pancreatic cancer.

This study also noted the presence of bacteria in bile, formerly thought to be sterile. In a study based on PDAC patients, Maekawa et.al., via genetic sequence analysis, found *Enterobacter* and *Enterococcus* spp were the major microbes.

The researchers cite prior research which identifies over 700 different bacterial species in the mouth. They acknowledge that most cannot be cultured as a means to study them. However, they cite other researchers who have studied both animal models and human subjects, and have verified the spread of oral microbes to pancreas via translocation or dissemination. Pathways are not discussed in these prior findings.

In their discussion of GI microbiota, the Fudan University cancer researchers say gut microbes can reach the pancreas through the circulatory system or the biliary/pancreatic duct, calling it transductal transmission.

And finally, the researchers note that the chemotherapy drug cyclophosphamide damages the intestinal mucus layer (likely they are referring to the MMM), allowing some gut bacteria (and potentially other microcontaminants) to enter the lymph nodes and spleen, where immune cells are then activated.

Vascular Microbiome and the Glycocalyx

Doctors Alison Clifford and Gary Hoffman reported in 2015 in *Current Opinion in Rheumatology* that blood vessels may not be sterile![3]

But we knew that already. Blood vessels cannot be "sterile" because they are one of the pathways for beneficial bacteria, harmful bacteria, cellular waste, and the MMM to circulate throughout your body.

In an article titled *Evidence for a vascular microbiome and its role in vessel health and disease*, Clifford and Hoffman discuss preliminary evidence that suggests that normal vessels may harbor microbes, where different communities of microbes may be present in inflammatory and noninflammatory large-blood vessel diseases.[3]

It's satisfying to see so many new studies questioning the impact of their new discoveries of a microbiome in various organs and systems.

In *An update on the microbiome in vasculitis* published in 2021 in *Current Opinion in Rheumatology*, researchers Shahna Tariq and Alison Clifford review studies describing the gastrointestinal, nasal, pulmonary, and vascular microbiomes.[4]

They reveal that dysbiosis and reduced microbial diversity are associated with patients with small, medium, and large blood vessel vasculitis.

Reitsma and Slaff teach that "The endothelial glycocalyx is a network of membrane-bound proteoglycans and glycoproteins, covering the endothelium luminally. Both endothelium- and plasma-derived soluble molecules integrate into this mesh. Over the past decade, insight has been gained into the role of the glycocalyx in vascular physiology and pathology, including mechanotransduction, hemostasis, signaling, and blood cell–vessel wall interactions. The contribution of the glycocalyx to diabetes, ischemia/reperfusion, and atherosclerosis is also reviewed. Experimental data from micro- and macro-circulation alludes to a vasculoprotective role for the glycocalyx. Assessing this possible role of the endothelial glycocalyx requires reliable visualization of this delicate layer, which is a great challenge. An overview is given of the various ways in which the endothelial glycocalyx has been visualized up to now, including first data from two-photon microscopic imaging."[5]

I believe that the glycocalyx is being interpreted as the structural portion of the MMM that can be seen with scanning electron microscopic imaging.

Liver / Lymph microbiome

Writing in the *Journal of Genetics* and *Genomics* in 2022, Chinese researchers identify a second connection between the gut microbiome and the liver.[6] The first connection was previously identified as the hepatic portal vein.

Performing metabolome comparison in blood and mesenteric lymph systems, the researchers note significantly shifted metabolites in serum and lymph. Thus, they have identified a second pathway for bacterial transport between the gut and liver.

Researchers summarize "establishment of the mesentery as a second route for the gut–liver axis expands our knowledge of mechanisms of gut microbial metabolites and gut–liver interactions in modulating host health and provides novel opportunities for the management of metabolic disorders."

Liver/Hepatic Microbiome

Thirty-eight New York researchers report that a robust hepatic microbiome exists in animal and human liver that is different from that of the host gastrointestinal tract.[7] Writing in *The Journal of Clinical Investigation* in 2022, these researchers provide significant evidence of the hepatic MMM, the effect of antibiotics on the hepatic MMM, the effect of changes in the gut and fecal transplants on the hepatic MMM, and discuss how hepatic immunity is dependent on the hepatic microbiome.

We knew this in general, but the researchers identified that oral antibiotics reduce liver immune cells by a remarkable approximately 90%, prevented antigen-presenting cell maturation, and reduced adaptive immunity.

Five distinct phyla were identified in the liver. They included *Bacteriodetes*, *Firmicutes*, *Proteobacteria*, and *Verrucomicrobia*. *Proteobacteria* represented an approximately 40-times greater portion of the liver microbiome compared with that of the gut.

Researchers postulated that the hepatic microbiome is selectively populated from the gut microbiome.

In comparison to different organs, the hepatic microbiome displayed characteristics most closely related to the pancreatic microbiome, versus the duodenum or gallbladder microbiomes.

Examining dynamics of the hepatic microbiome, researchers noted that the microbiome varies with age, sex, and environment.

The researchers studied effects of oral antibiotics on the hepatic microbiome. They found that selective oral antibiotic treatment with metronidazole, vancomycin, or combination neomycin/ampicillin each resulted in lower *Bacteriodetes* similar to that seen with broad-spectrum antibiotics. In addition, decreased alpha-diversity richness was shown. Alpha diversity describes the bacterial species diversity within a community at a small or local scale.

Researchers describe the hepatic microbiome as bacterial communities within the tissue and described their role in leukocyte recruitment and activation.

The article further elucidates distinct community identities in gut versus liver and central versus peripheral hepatic microbial communities. They write that this is consistent with the branched segmented distribution of the biliary tree and its interstitum and portal venous circulation. Thus they have postulated that there are at least two plausible modes of translocation of the MMM.

Researchers at the University of Copenhagen, Denmark, examined the hepatic and blood microbiomes in healthy lean and obese humans in a paper published in JHEP Reports in 2021.[8]

Their report established microbial diversity in biopsies from the obese group compared to the healthy group. Thus, they propose that changes in the liver microbiome could be an additional risk factor for non-alcoholic fatty liver disease (NAFLD).

Researchers also note that differences in the liver microbiome between obese and lean individuals are not reflected in the blood microbiome. In so doing, they have differentiated between liver and blood microbiomes.

Placenta Microbiome

I was very excited after reading an article when it was published in 2014 by researchers at Baylor College of Medicine in Houston, Texas.[9] **Another nail in the coffin for medical dogma. For, the placenta was supposed to be sterile, and babies were supposed to be sterile before they are born.**

If medicine is so naïve about how babies develop in the womb and their condition when they are born, especially by Cesarian section, what do we really know about the human condition?

In this article, researchers describe the human placental microbiome.[9] They demonstrate that the placental microbiome is a low-abundance and metabolically rich microbiome. **It contains nonpathogenic commensal bacteria of the *Firmicutes*, *Tenericutes*, *Proteobacteria*, *Bacteriodetes*, and *Fusobacteria* phyla. The placental microbiome was most like the nonpregnant human oral microbiome. Ponder that!**

For their study, researchers sampled the placental microbiome of 320 subjects, all women (just checking to be sure you are paying attention). The characteristics of the placental microbiome were then compared to other human body sites including the oral, skin, nasal, vaginal, and gut microbiomes from nonpregnant women who served as controls.

I find this fascinating on many levels. It is disruptive to medical dogma regarding sterility of the placenta and the notion that a baby is sterile before it is born. There is no direct pathway from the mouth to the placenta, whose microbiomes are most alike. We would assume that these microbiota originate in the mouth, but that is not confirmed. It seems obvious that the direct pathway is not the GI tract, leaving the bloodstream, lymph system, and interstitial space as possibilities. And finally, my MMM hypothesis predicted this and so many other discoveries.

Fetal Microbiome

A 2019 study in humans and mice demonstrated that a fetus has its own gut microbiome.[10] Experimenters also verified that the fetal microbiome is transmitted from the mother during fetal development. These findings open the door to interventions during gestation to stimulate the fetal microbiome when an early birth is anticipated, to help the baby grow briskly and be better equipped to tolerate early life infection threat. The study was published in the journal JCI *Insight*.

"Our study provides strong proof that a complex microbiome is transmitted from the mother to the fetus," says senior author Patrick Seed, MD, PhD, Associate Chief Research Officer of Basic Sciences at Stanley Manne Children's Research Institute at Ann & Robert H. Lurie Children's Hospital of Chicago, and Research Professor of Pediatrics, Microbiology and Immunology at Northwestern University Feinberg School of Medicine. "Unlike other studies relying only on next generation DNA sequencing, we validated our sequencing results with microscopy and culture techniques, to resolve a decades long controversy about the existence of a fetal microbiome. Now we can pursue ways to boost the development of fetal immune system and metabolism by stimulating mom's microbiome. Our findings point to many promising opportunities for much earlier intervention to prevent future disease."

Not only do the researchers establish the existence of the fetal microbiome, but they propose that pathways exist within the mother for bacteria to be transported from the gut of the mom to the fetal gut. Then they suggest the value of the fetal gut microbiome in the growth and development of the infant.

Urethral and Bladder Microbiome

In 2020, researchers at George Washington Schools of Medicine and Public Health in Washington DC reported on their exploration of the tools they used to identify differences between the human bladder and urethral microbiomes.[11]

In their introduction, the researchers suggest that medical dogma holds that the urine of healthy asymptomatic individuals is sterile. They then disproved the dogma and began to identify unique bacterial communities in the bladder and urethra.

They evaluated a small cohort of six healthy women and 14 men using urine cultures and 16S ribosomal RNA gene amplification sequencing. 16S DNA sequencing is a new method to identify bacteria by analyzing its DNA. All bacteria identified by culture were also identified by 16S amplification, but the opposite did not hold true.

Lactobacillus and *Streptococcus* were the most abundant species. The ratio of the nine predominant bacterial genera differed between the urethra and bladder, and between men and women.

Researchers at the Heimholtz Centre for Infection Research in Braunschweig, Germany published interesting results in 2017.[12]

They found a microbiome community of 497 taxonomic units (different bacterial strains) in human urine.

They showed that orally applied antibiotic medication (metronidazole) significantly reduced diversity and the relative abundance of various pathogenic bacteria, but increased other pathogenic bacteria in the urinary tract of men and women.

They noted that bacterial vaginosis (BV) has a 60% recurrence rate in 12 months after treatment with the standard of care antibiotic metronidazole. Current standard of care only provides for destruction; it does not provide for restoration of the MMM. It's great to see this effect of incomplete antibiotic treatment (lacking in repopulation of the microbiome) elucidated.

Researchers concluded that oral use of metronidazole in women with BV caused massive changes in urine microbiota composition, BUT IT DID NOT RESTORE A HEALTHY BACTERIAL COMMUNITY. The medical community leaves restoration of a healthy microbiome to chance, after they have destroyed the microbiome with antibiotics.

Thyroid Microbiome

In 2021, researchers in the Departments of Surgery, Surgical Oncology, and Pathology at the First Affiliated Hospital of Nanchang University, China published a study *Alterations of thyroid microbiota across different thyroid microhabitats in patients with thyroid carcinoma.*[13]

They performed 16s rRNA gene sequencing using tumor tissues and biopsies from matched peritumor (the area around a tumor) tissues from 30 patients to understand the thyroid microbiome.

Researchers found that richness and diversity of thyroid microbiome were lower in thyroid cancer tumor samples than in matched peritumor tissues. They also concluded that a higher abundance of Sphingomonas was correlated with lymph node metastasis.

Researchers also noted other studies which observed a decrease in microbiome diversity in patients with lung cancer and gastric cancer.

Brain Microbiome

It seems that scientists and patients alike are reluctant to perform brain biopsies in order to study the microbiome in healthy brains. I don't blame them.

Just like so many other organs, medical dogma held that the brain was sterile, or that bacteria in the brain were thought to be signs of disease.

In an accidental finding, where scientists were looking for differences in the brains of people with and without schizophrenia using electron microscopy, the scientists kept finding mysterious rod-shaped objects.[14] These rod-shaped objects were found in all 34 postmortem human brains examined in the study.

Using genetic sequencing the researchers discovered that most of the brain microbes were from groups of bacteria typically found in the human gut.

Scientists at the University of Birmingham, Alabama then tried to determine if these beneficial bacteria, known as *Firmicutes*, *Proteobacteria*, and *Bacteriodetes* were seen because of contamination of all 34 brains. They concluded that neither their samples nor procedures were contaminated.

These 2018 findings raise the possibility that the brain may have a microbiome! And suggest the question of how live, healthy bacteria are translocated from the gut to the brain or vice-versa?

In this review, it was mentioned that the brain would then join an onslaught of previously considered sterile organs, such as women's fallopian tubes and ovaries and men's testes. All of these also have microbiomes, blasting the dogma of sterility throughout the human body and raising the broad questions of where and for what purpose a microbiome exists in all these organs in the body. Hint, this thinking suggests the value of MMM Theory.

Cartilage Microbiome

Rheumatology researchers in France posed the questions: What is a microbiome doing in cartilage? How did it get there? How does the microbiome affect cartilage in osteoarthritis? And why is the microbiome different in the hip and knee?

These researchers seemed to infer the question, what is the gut microbiome doing in cartilage? And how does the gut microbiome relocating to cartilage effect osteoarthritis?

They elucidate that trafficing of DNA microbiota to the joints is the rule, not an exception. And they go on to cite studies that the blood of healthy humans is not sterile – it contains bacteria, i.e.: a plasma microbiome.

Writing in 2019, these researchers express that the gut microbiome was recently found in human cartilage.[15] It differs between individuals with OA and those who do not present with OA symptoms.

They ponder the means of relocation of the microbiome into cartilage because the average pore size in the cartilage extracellular matrix is 6 nm, but the average size of most bacteria

ranges from 100 to 4,000 nm. Perhaps, they say, microbial DNA was stored in bone marrow and migrated to the adjacent cartilage. This is a predicament because cartilage itself does not have blood vessels, nerves, or lymphatics in the middle and deep zones.

And yet we recall how surprised the scientists were who discovered an advanced vascular system in bones just eight years ago. This vascular system in bones finally explained how stem cells and immune cells formed in bone marrow quickly travel to an injury elsewhere in the body.

Prosthetic joint infection (PJI) is a devastating complication following arthroplasty. Researchers attempted to clarify risk factors and microbiology of PJI. They established that the most frequently found microorganisms are found in the skin microbiome. These researchers postulated that microorganisms get into the joint and infect the prosthesis during and after joint replacement procedures. However, recent studies have shown bacteria may be present in the joint even before the first incision, suggesting the existence of a joint microbiome. Therefore, researchers sought to quantify the bacterial composition from different knee conditions.[16]

Vaginal Microbiome

European and Israeli researchers explored the vaginal microbiome in a 2022 paper.[17,18]

They detected over 20 species of *lactobacilli* bacteria but found that in most women the vagina is dominated by a single species.

Characteristics of the vagina include a pH level less than 4.5 (acidic), which is unique compared with other mammals which have a greater mixture of bacterial species and a pH closer to 7 (neutral). **So once again, the warning to avoid alkaline water in your vagina for any reason – it will neutralize the pH and reduce the protective effects of the acidic environment against STDs and other infections. In addition, it could alter the natural bacterial mix of the vaginal microbiome.**

The researchers describe the complexity of the vaginal milieu – which bathes the *Lactobacillus* and other organisms in a complex mix of fluids, sluffing epithelial cells, secretions from the cervix, and inflammatory cells.

They describe the vaginal microbiome as a dynamic ecosystem, fluctuating throughout a woman's life. These changes are influenced by hormones, glycogen content, menstrual cycle, vaginal pH, and immune responses.

The researchers concluded their study by identifying approximately 16,000 unique bacterial families per community in the vagina, compared with almost 400,000 in the mouth.

Mitochondrial Microbiome

This discussion is most interesting. This information is based on a 2017 article titled *The Microbiome-Mitochondrion Connection: Common Ancestries, Common Mechanisms, Common Goals*, published by two researchers in Singapore and Illinois in mSystems, a journal of the American Society for Microbiology.[19]

In the 1960s, modern cellular biology established that there is a shared evolution between bacteria and mitochondria. Human mitochondria are descendants of primordial aerobic bacteria that entered into a synergistic partnership with ancient anaerobic microbes.

So, mitochondria, the powerhouses of a cell, are descendants of bacteria! Excluding our microbiome, we are partially bacteria or descended from bacteria! Look that up in your family tree!

Other research I found cites an average of 2,500 mitochondria per human cell. Not only does the human microbiome vastly outnumber the cells in our bodies, but the descendants of bacteria – the mitochondria organelles - vastly outnumber the cells in our bodies.

The researchers point out that nutrient metabolism is a function of both the microbiome and mitochondria. Of three key microbiome metabolites – short-chain fatty acids, urolithins, and lactate – butyrate (a short chain fatty acid) and urolithin A enhance microbial diversity.

The authors identified that probiotic supplementation with *Lactobacillus plantarum* exerts beneficial effects over muscle performance, oxidative capacity, and increased colonic short-chain fatty acids. Exercise helps to quench systemic inflammation, increase fatty acid oxidation, promote mitochondrial biogenesis, and promote microbiome diversity.

This finding of MMM Theory research suggests a new way to support muscle and athletic performance and slow osteopenia.

Plasma Microbiome

In a beautiful article titled *The Healthy Human Blood Microbiome: Fact or Fiction?* researchers report that medical dogma holds that human blood and the vascular system are sterile.[20] The detection of bacteria in blood has been consistently (naively) interpreted as a sign of infection.

However, evidence to the contrary is steadily accumulating, report the researchers writing in a 2019 article in *Frontiers in Cellular Infection Microbiology*.

Researchers evaluated 19 studies which demonstrated evidence of a microbiome in human blood.

Of note, Whittle et.al. (2018) demonstrated that the blood-microbiome closely resembles the skin and oral microbiomes. It differs substantially from the intestinal microbiome.

They write that the healthy human blood microbiome (HBM) is highly dynamic. Of course, that makes it so much more difficult to define it, count it, and identify a "normal" HBM, as current medical dogma tries so hard to do. This too means there will be no silver bullet cure for a dysbiotic human blood microbiome. Dominant blood-borne bacterial phyla include *Proteobacteria*, *Actinobacteria*, *Firmicutes* and *Bacteriodetes*.

Paisse et.al. (2016) identified primarily white blood cells and platelets as the location of the blood microbiome of healthy patients. However, some bacteria reside in red blood cells and thrive in this nutrient-rich environment. Staphylococcus aureus can utilize iron in red blood cells as a nutrient source. What does this mean when we discuss iron-rich or poor blood and its physiologic impact on human energy levels?

A limited number of studies have explored the relationship of the human blood microbiome and its role in disease. Diabetes, pancreatitis, cardiovascular and liver disease have been related to changes in the human blood microbiome.

In an editorial, researchers in Beijing, China commented on the plasma microbiome in patients with Systemic Lupus Erythematosus (SLE).[21] They reviewed a 2022 *Journal of Rheumatology* study where James and colleagues examined the plasma and intestinal microbiomes of female patients with SLE and healthy controls.

They found that the plasma microbial diversity was significantly decreased in patients with SLE as compared to healthy controls. They found that the intestinal microbiome in these two patient populations did not differ significantly. This observation highlighted the relationship of the plasma microbiome to SLE, whereas the intestinal microbiome did not seem to be correlated with SLE.

Reseachers at McMaster University, Ontario, Canada published the results of their work in September 2022. They used blood cells to create a trojan horse delivery mechanism for drugs. These blood cells were emptied. Strong and dangerous antibiotics such as Polymyxin B were then encapsulated in the liposome – the blood cell membrane. The membrane was then coated with antibodies, allowing it to flow through the vascular system and stick to target bacteria, such as E. Coli. This is a novel use of the blood microbiome for targeted drug delivery. It is further described in Chapter 2 – You Are Being Poisoned.

Skin Microbiome

You've always heard that vitamin D is produced in your skin when it is exposed to sunlight. Does any of that make sense? Your skin just creates vitamin D from sunlight? Skin makes more vitamin D if you live closer to the equator. It makes less if you live further from hot sunlight or cover your skin with clothes or chemicals such as in commercial sunscreen. It makes less if you stay indoors, or are elderly and stay indoors.

Vitamin D is produced by a process of fermentation in and on your skin. Bacteria in your skin are triggered by sunlight to produce vitamin D. Just as in your gut, your skin tissue does not perform fermentation; the bacteria or microbiome in your gut ferments foods you have eaten.

New research establishes the size of the skin surface as 30 square meters (323 square feet). That means someone 6 feet tall would have skin that when laid flat would need a belt or a necklace that is 53 feet long!

Rather than looking at the visible surface area of the skin, this is calculated by establishing the surface area of the skin that is exposed to bacteria. This new surface area measurement takes into account the surface area of follicles to yield an area about 10 times larger than previously thought. This surface area, invisible to the naked eye, is likely where bacterial fermentation of vitamin D occurs. A further discussion once again defying anatomical dogma that the skin surface area is smaller than that of the GI tract and lungs will be found in Chapter 8 – Skin Microbiome.

Conclusion

From a sampling of scientific literature published by researchers around the world, we have highlighted that a microbiome exists in and surrounding almost every organ in the human body. Plus, it exists in organs in a developing fetus.

Researchers have confirmed the vascular and lymph systems as pathways for bacteria to travel throughout the body.

Still much is to be learned about the microbial mucosal milieu (MMM).

CHAPTER FOUR

INTRODUCTION TO AUTOIMMUNE DISEASE, INFLAMMATION, AND THE MMM

Any discussion of autoimmune disease is by its nature long, complex, and controversial, for 100+ diseases have been categorized as autoimmune. They each present in a different part or parts of the body. They each are diagnosed and treated by a different medical specialty.

However, one thing they all have in common is that your allopathic doctor will eventually admit that modern medicine does not know the root cause of the "disease."

The root cause of "Autoimmune Disease" and inflammation are perhaps the most profound insights proposed by MMM Theory, for once you know what is causing the "disease," you can treat the cause rather than the symptoms. Or worse in the long-term, treat the body's protective mechanisms. At least now you will understand the imbalance you are provoking when you need to "treat" or stop the body's natural protective mechanisms that are trying to fight the disease.

I put "autoimmune disease" in quotes because I do not believe these symptoms represent diseases.

To cut to the chase, I believe these symptoms, however serious and debilitating they are, represent the body's natural response to contaminants that have entered the body and cause a protective reaction by the body. Rather than the body attacking itself, the body is attacking the microcontaminants. The tissue surrounding the accumulation of these microcontaminants then suffers from collateral damage.

For example, if you cut yourself, the area around the cut becomes inflamed, not just the cut tissue.

How do these microcontaminants congregate in a particular part of the body and reach a tipping point where we notice the body attacking these molecules?

They accumulate in the body, and in a particular organ, as a result of a breach or weakness in the MMM and possibly prior injury or genetic weakness affecting that body part.

The MMM naturally acts to protect the body from allopathically known and unknown microcontaminants. It functions in any and every part of the body.

One of the body's most effective responses is inflammation. Inflammation is the body's response to the presence of environmental contaminants and disruptive forces in an attempt to isolate and remove the toxins. The U.S. National Institute of Health, National Institute of Environmental Health Sciences attributes inflammation to many factors, such as environmental chemicals, injuries, pathogens like bacteria, viruses, or fungi, and radiation.[1]

Thus, MMM theory also propounds a primary cause of inflammation and pain.

However, we know there are other causes of inflammation and pain, such as the response to a physical injury, like hitting your thumb with a hammer.

While we are saving major discussions about the gastrointestinal tract for our second book, for purposes of discussing autoimmune disease, I will focus on the intestines. That is where MMM theory was initially developed due to my proctitis, later diagnosed as ulcerative colitis "autoimmune disease."

Figure 1

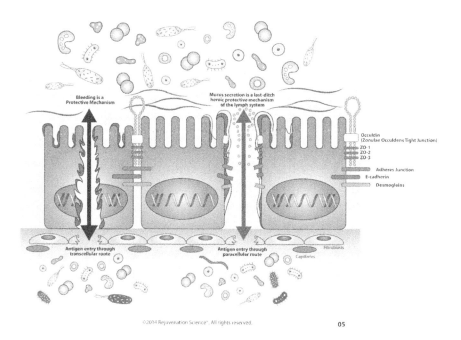

Figure 1 shows three adjacent epithelial cells in the large intestine. At the top of the picture is the bolus – the flow of food, nutrients, liquid, digested food, bacteria, contaminants, dead cells, and waste material through the intestines.

You can see that the epithelial cells are red, inflamed, disrupted, and there are breaks in and between cells. Fibroblasts which line the inner surface of the cells are damaged in places. Capillaries are exposed to nutrients, but also to materials which should not have breached the epithelial tissue.

We will focus on the wavy lines floating above the epithelial tissue. These wavy lines represent the Mucosal Microbial Milieu (MMM).

The cause of all this cellular and intestinal dysbiosis is a weakness or breach in the MMM.

The inflammation and redness is caused as the body reacts to the contaminants that do not belong in contact with the epithelial tissue or surface of the intestine.

These contaminants may include hydrocarbons, plastics, BPA, parabens, toluene, benzene, styrene, phthalates), cellular waste material, non-buffered hydrochloric acid from the stomach or the opposite, too much alkalinity from overproduction of bile, as well as irritating or harmful bacteria and viruses.

SYMPTOMS

All of the symptoms that an ulcerative colitis sufferer experiences represent the body's reaction to these microcontaminants that do not belong where they have entered. The symptoms range from mild to severe, always present as inflammation, and include:

GI upset – colloquially called upset stomach. An upset stomach is very vague and doesn't isolate the cause to any particular condition.

Diarrhea – is the body's attempt to clear microcontaminants or toxins from the colon. We all know it is effective and unpleasant.

Constipation – alterations in the serotonergic receptor activity, imbalance of parasympathetic and sympathetic tone, which contribute to further irritation of the gastrointestinal lumen. Additionally, slow GI transit time becomes the breeding ground for increased toxin production and reabsorption of metabolites, toxins, and waste products.

Poor appetite – provides less bolus to enable healing of the intestinal wall. Unfortunately, it also has the effect of decreasing nutrients available for healing. In altered physiological states, the need for increased nutrient status to shift from disruption to homeostasis is very common. Poor appetite can contribute to nutrient deficits that perpetuate pathophysiology.

Abdominal pain – signaling the body to rest. This is one of many measures of patient status and can be used as a metric for aggravation arising from interventional therapies, or a shift in the wellness status, whether driven by food, inflammatory process, ulceration, poor digestion, or infectious processes, or beneficial and harmful bacterial conflict.

Fatigue/fever – fever may arise in response to infection or cytokine storm, while fatigue may also arise from disrupted sleep, toxin reabsorption from the GI tract into circulation, and even shifts in thyroid status (thyroid dysregulation arising from a decrease in T3 and increase in reverse T3), or simply poor nutritional status.

Elevated antibodies – to fight infection

GI ulcerations – represent damage to the intestinal wall. They are like open wounds in your intestines and are very uncomfortable. **Uninformed diets that include roughage can exacerbate the distress of GI ulcerations or raw GI epithelial tissue. Roughage can include raw and cooked vegetables, especially corn and greens. Nuts and seeds can be physically scratchy in an irritated intestine. Spices can either trigger healing or irritate the intestinal surface. Sparkling drinks can exacerbate gas or bloating.**

GI bleeding – an extreme defensive measure to clean and stabilize the damage to the intestinal wall. Bleeding is a sign of serious damage and dysfunction of the intestinal wall. The loss of red blood cells results in increased nutritional demand to replace lost blood. Additionally, the disruption of the epithelial lining of the GI tract may contribute to increased susceptibility to secondary microbial infection and enhanced risk of pathogens entering central circulation.

GI cramping – an extreme defensive measure to clean and clear the contaminants and toxicants from the GI tract.

Bowel urgency – a further extreme defensive measure to clean and clear contaminants and toxicants from the GI tract. This is when you have to go BAD and FAST. It leads to another syndrome called bathroom seeking, where the patient tries to always know where the nearest AVAILABLE bathroom is. It is sometimes debilitating and difficult to work, travel, or do anything in public. I've had to use a porta-potty at a construction site a block away from my doctor's office because the office was too far away to make it in time. I also carried a foldup camping toilet in the trunk of my car for some peace of mind.

GI mucus – one of your body's more extreme defensive measures to protect the damaged epithelial tissue from the bolus flowing by to allow the tissue to heal or repair itself. Throughout the body, mucus is often a marker for either infection or inflammatory processes.

Polyps – a longer-term extreme defensive measure to patch the damaged tissue. Polyps are markers for damaged tissue, which includes DNA damage to that tissue. These may mark increased risk of pathogenic change over time, including at times increased risk of carcinogenic changes.

Colorectal cancer – the result of long-term DNA damage to tissue in the colon and rectum.

DIAGNOSIS

Your general practitioner or gastroenterologist will diagnose you on a spectrum of:

Indigestion

Food poisoning

Heartburn or GERD (Gastroesophageal Reflux Disease) occurs when stomach acid repeatedly flows back into the tube connecting your mouth and stomach (esophagus). This backwash (acid reflux) can irritate and damage the lining of your esophagus.

Irritable Bowel Syndrome (IBS)

Inflammatory Bowel Disease (IBD)

   Colitis

Ulcerative Colitis

Crohn's Disease

Diverticulitis

Pouchitis – an inflammation of the pouch that was created post pan colectomy (removal of the entire colon) surgery. I was diagnosed with this after exposure to high levels of mold for 1 ½ years. In my case, mold was the environmental contaminant that accumulated at my weakest link (weakened by genetics and damaged by long-term inflammation and surgery) and triggered an inflammatory immune response.

MMM Theory suggests a diagnosis of damaged and dysfunctional MMM, presenting as any of the above diagnoses and likely comorbidities (other symptoms, such as brain fog, ADHD, nerve issues, joint issues, and more). It is fundamentally important to not just pursue symptoms, rather address the underlying cause of each individual sign and symptoms. As stated in Latin, **Tolle Causam, which means** identify and treat the origin of the dysfunction. As, Dr. Meletis shares with his patients:

> "Indeed, disharmony within the body begets dysfunction, and dysfunction begets disharmony."

TREATMENTS

Standard IBS and IBD treatments may include:

Dietary alterations, looking for food sensitivities. Common culprits found are sensitivities to milk products, wheat, and spicy foods. Sometimes removal of these foods from your diet reduces symptoms, but it does not address the cause of the problem. Milk product sensitivity is usually only cow's milk products, such as cheese, yogurt, batter (such as used on fried chicken or other dredged products), flavorings, whey, creamer, sour cream, smoothies, chocolate, and more. A hyper-vigilant immune system that is further triggered by immune-reactive food antigens or microbes perpetuates a state of "disease."

Stress reduction. Stress exacerbates and contributes to many diseases. However, by itself, I don't think it is a primary cause of an autoimmune disease such as UC. It has been noted though that stress does lower IgA levels within the body, particularly important in inflammatory bowel disease and other mucous membrane presentations. Indeed sufficient secretory IgA is needed to confer what Dr. Meletis refers to as "water proofing" or "Scotch guarding" the mucous membranes from infectious and noxious agents.

Anti-diarrheal drugs. "Let's treat or try to stop the body's protective mechanism, which is trying to clear contaminants from the intestines," say too many people who are attempting a quick fix at the expense of a long-term remedy. In the presence of endotoxins or toxic substances, use of anti-motility interventions can further tissue damage and total body burden and can risk the individual's global well-being. There is a time and place to break the vicious cycle of chronic or debilitating diarrhea, yet only after thorough clinical consideration and appropriate testing identifying the etiology for the rapid bowel transit time.

Antibiotic drugs. These are helpful if an imbalance of harmful bacteria exist. However, leaving a bacterial wasteland behind, possibly throughout the entire body depending on the specificity of the antibiotic drug, is potentially harmful in the long term. Thus, it is critical to repopulate the bacterial milieu with beneficial bacteria for long-term health. See my analogy in Chapter 2, where a farmer clears his land and leaves it for opportunistic plants like weeds to grow back.

Corticosteroids. These drugs have a long history of use before the creation of biological medications, as they lower immune and inflammatory responses. They also contribute to catabolic (decreased healing) in contrast to anabolism (building up of simple molecules to generate complex molecules, such as amino acids to proteins).

Immunosuppressant drugs such as methotrexate. Immunosuppressant medications can contribute to dysregulation of the MMM, increase the risk of pathogenic infection, and alter immune system competence to maintain broad diversity and micro-ecology locally and globally. In the case of methotrexate, its direct effect on folate can contribute to increased risk of leaky gut, diminished restorative/healing processes, and enhanced risk of not only leaky gut, but also disruption of other microbiomes that when further perceived by immune surveillance can aggravate the individual's susceptibility to other disharmonious processes.

Biologics: infliximab, Humira, Entyvio. The list of side effects of this category of medications point to a myriad of changes in the physiological processes. Thus judicious use, with appropriate weighing of benefits and risk is important. Indeed, clinical consideration of additional interventional therapeutics to mitigate the side effect profile seems prudent – much like folate is monitored and typically prescribed along with methotrexate.

Other standard treatments. These include polypectomy, surgical resection, and surgical removal.

MMM Theory suggests the following IBS and IBD treatments:

Remove precipitating factors – reduce exposure to environmental contaminants that harm the MMM.These include:

- Herbicides and pesticides in non-organic food
- Herbicides and pesticides used around the house or at work
- Antibiotics (as much as possible)
- Cleaning and sanitizing solution residue
- Chlorine in drinking water, bath, and shower water
- Living near hydrocarbon centers such as oil fields, tar pits, major freeways or highways, airports, plastics industry, other industrial centers, fuel/gas stations, attached garage without ventilation, and poorly vented natural gas or propane use.

CURRENT IBS and IBD ETIOLOGY / EXPLANATIONS

Some explanations include:

1. Immune system reacts abnormally
2. Immune system attacks the gastrointestinal tract
3. White blood cell proliferation
4. Or the truthful one: We really don't know the cause

IBS and IBD PROGNOSIS WITH ALOPATHIC TREATMENT

Possible outcomes of allopathic treatment include:

- Periods of remission
- Unpredictable recurrence
- General worsening of symptoms over time
- Higher risk of cancer
- Eventual surgical intervention

PROGRESSION OF GI DISEASE

Figure 2

From healthy to mild irritation to severe "auto-immune" disease:

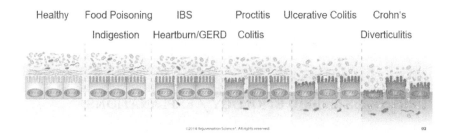

- Decreasing integrity of microbial mucosal milieu resulting in increasing symptomology.
- Commensurate decreasing health of GI epithelial cells (the mucosal membrane).
- Increasing progression of contaminants entering local tissue, bloodstream, and lymphatic system.

- Increasing severity of disease diagnosis.

The wavy lines represent the MMM. The MMM acts as the protective barrier between all that flows through the intestines (the bolus) and the intestinal lining of the tissue. It protects the delicate epithelial tissue, ferments food, and passes nutrients to the tissue. It also passes waste material from the tissue back into the flow through the colon and rectum. Imagine the sophistication of managing the flow of nutrients (incoming) with waste (outgoing) through the same GI tube.

How does this mess with your paradigm regarding sanitary? In other words, to know that nutrients/food for your body are moving along with waste from your body throughout your body. Too much information would be the knowledge that your drinking water and your poop flow simultaneously through the same tubes in your body. This occurs in the GI tract, in your bloodstream, your lymph system, your glymphatic system, and the interstitial space between cells.

MMM Theory proposed mechanism of action is the sophistication of the diversity of bacteria making up your MMM. And we're only just beginning to appreciate the MMM, because we will identify its function in all the other circulatory systems in your body – your vascular/blood system, your lymph system, your glymphatic system, your sinuses, and the interstitial spaces in your body.

All these flows allow contaminants to enter and facilitate their removal from your body, with the result being health or disease – most likely identified as autoimmune disease, where the body attacks contaminants that breach the MMM. The body does not attack healthy tissue, though there is collateral damage to healthy tissue, which presents with inflammation and many other symptoms.

Your GI tract can't be impermeable like a plastic, glass, or metal container that can hold hydrochloric acid and protein/tissue digesting enzymes. Sounds like the stomach, doesn't it? Have you ever thought about what keeps the hydrochloric acid and protein digestive enzymes from digesting your stomach tissue? Yet your stomach is not impermeable plastic or glass. The answer is the MMM.

Nor can your GI tract be porous like a sieve that spreads fertilizer to nourish crops. Your GI tract must provide a very sophisticated semi-permeable membrane that "intelligently" lifts nutrients from the bolus and deposits waste into the bolus. There is no point of demarcation in your intestines where up to that point nutrients flow and after that red line, waste flows.

I'm suggesting that it is bacteria in the MMM that provide sanitary barriers inside your body. This is a lot to think about, because on the surface it is so contrary to conventional dogma. Yet we cite so many new studies that demonstrate exactly these concepts I envisioned in 2014.

Now back to Figure 2. As the MMM sustains damage and becomes less effective, the damaged MMM allows microcontaminants to enter the epithelial tissue, these contaminants damage the tissue, decreasing the health of epithelial cells that make up the intestinal tissue membrane. Subsequently the contaminants enter your bloodstream and lymph system. Figure 2 shows the protective effect of the MMM and subsequently more severe diagnosis as the health of the MMM is degraded by environmental contaminants.

INFLAMMATION

Inflammation plays a key role in diseases classified as autoimmune disease.

There are two primary classifications of inflammation – acute and chronic.

The four cardinal signs of acute inflammation first noted by the Greek physician Celsus about 200 A.D. are redness, heat, swelling and pain. In injured tissues, blood vessels widen and blood flow surges, causing redness and heat. The walls of inflamed blood vessels become more porous, allowing inflammatory cells, protein, and fluid to leak into tissues, creating swelling and putting painful pressure on nerve endings.

Chronic inflammation is damaging when it occurs in healthy tissue or lasts too long. Here it is silent or hidden, but is more likely than acute inflammation to cause DNA damage.

Beyond the obvious symptoms, the presence of cytokines and other inflammatory markers demonstrate the presence of inflammation.

Inflammation is the body's response to the presence of environmental contaminants in an attempt to isolate and remove the toxins. The U.S. National Institute of Health, National Institute of Environmental Health Sciences, attributes inflammation to many factors, such as environmental chemicals, injuries, pathogens like bacteria, viruses, or fungi, and radiation.[2]

NIEHS writes that inflammation plays a key role in many diseases, some of which are becoming more common and severe. Chronic inflammatory diseases contribute to more than half of deaths worldwide![3]

NIEHS writes that increasing evidence suggests environmental factors contribute to chronic inflammation. A review of scientific literature conducted by NIEHS-funded researchers affiliated with the National Toxicology Program found that the environment plays a role in inflammation in both positive and negative ways, such as:[3]

- **Environmental chemicals** – The federal Toxicology in the 21st Century, or Tox21, program shows how chemicals we commonly encounter may alter molecular pathways that underlie inflammation.[4]
- **Nutrition** – Diets high in refined grains, alcohol, and processed foods can alter gut microbiota and lead to intestinal and immune changes.
- **Microbiome** – Studies of various microbiome imbalances and disease states show connections to inflammation.
- **Social and cultural changes** – Disrupted sleep patterns, psychosocial stress, artificial light, and other factors influence the immune system.
- **Developmental origins** – Childhood obesity, psychological stress, exposure to microbes in infancy, and prenatal conditions are linked to inflammation.
- **Physical activity** – When skeletal muscles contract, they release proteins that can reduce inflammation throughout the body.

HIGHLIGHTS

We have now posited the cause of inflammation, established the cause of acute and chronic diseases, established how to prevent the causes of inflammation, and thus how to prevent or treat acute and chronic diseases that present as inflammatory diseases.

Figure 3

Inflammation and Cancer Risk

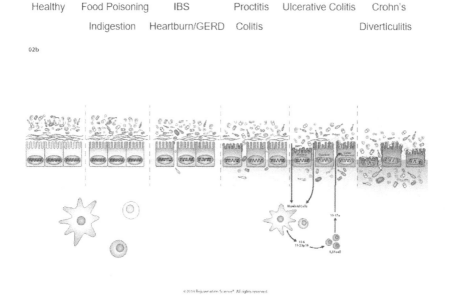

Long term inflammation increases the risk of cellular DNA damage. Increased DNA damage increases the risk of cancer.

Because of my increased risk of colon cancer, my gastroenterologist recommended that I have a colonoscopy annually. I tended to do it biannually for about 25 years. They're not fun. It's actually the preparation that is the worst part, not the procedure itself. Preparation involves clearing your intestines of everything. It is a washing process which uses a salt solution to cause your intestines to reverse the flow of water in the tissue. Rather than water becoming urine, the gallons of water you drink stay in your intestines and just flush them out.

Limitations of Colonoscopy

Figure 4

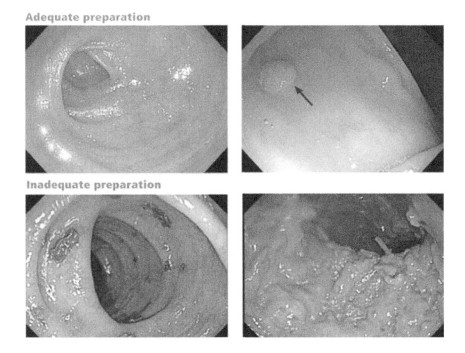

Adequate preparation

Inadequate preparation

Photo source: mesotheliomacancer1.info

The goal of a colonoscopy, proctoscopy, or sigmoidoscopy is to visually examine the surface of the colon or rectum. GI tissue cannot be seen when it is covered with bolus or the MMM. In a GI inspection, practitioners are blind to the value of the MMM – the floating protective layer throughout your GI tract. In fact, your surgeon has had you wash it away so that they can see the tissue!

Colonoscopy prep is a very good cleanse! However, it also flushes out your MMM so that your gastroenterologist or colorectal surgeon can see the endothelial tissue, the surface of your large intestines. This methodology allows your gastroenterologist to see any damage that has occurred to the surface. It also allows him or her to take biopsies for a pathologist to microscopically examine.

Figure 5

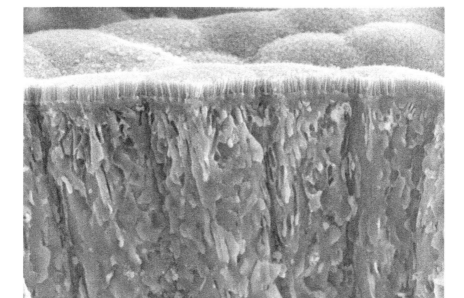

Microvilli in the small intestine, colored freeze-fracture scanning electron micrograph (SEM). The microvilli (across upper center) are tiny finger-like projections from the cells lining the interior wall of the small intestine. In this fracture view, the interiors of the underlying cells are also seen. The lining of the small intestine is thrown into numerous small folds called villi, which increase the surface area available for the absorption of nutrients from food. The microvilli on each cell increase this surface area yet further, making absorption highly efficient. Magnification x2800 when printed 10cm wide.

But see how "clean" the surface of the microvilli are. The MMM is nowhere to be seen.

Most bacteria are 0.2µm (micron) in diameter and 2–8µm (micron) in length. Bacterial cells are about one-tenth the size of eukaryotic cells. To see bacteria in this picture, the magnification would need to be increased 100 times, from x2800 to x280,000. To see microcontaminant molecules as I posit, magnification would need to be x1,000,000,000.

Science has no tools that can view the living mucosal milieu, nor has anyone trained in the field conceptualized the components, function, or value of the mucosal milieu, whose dysfunction is the root cause of most GI disease.

A scanning electron microscope is a type of electron microscope that produces images of a sample by scanning the surface with a focused beam of electrons. The electrons interact with atoms in the sample, producing various signals that contain information about the surface topography and composition of the sample.

The low end of the magnification range for an SEM is typically on the order of 20X to 50X. The maximum magnification is generally determined by the size of the electron beam and can be as high as one million ($10^{\wedge}6$).

Molecules commonly used as building blocks for organic synthesis have a dimension of a few angstroms (Å) to several dozen Å, or around one billionth of a meter. A microscope that can show something magnified 1,000,000 (million) times will not show anything that needs 1,000,000,000 (billion) magnification.

Did you ever think that your doctor and medical researchers are essentially blind to the cause of inflammation and the diseases they identify?

Practitioners admit to not understanding the cause of GI dysfunction, and diagnose the body's natural immune response to contaminants as the cause of GI disease.

Figure 6

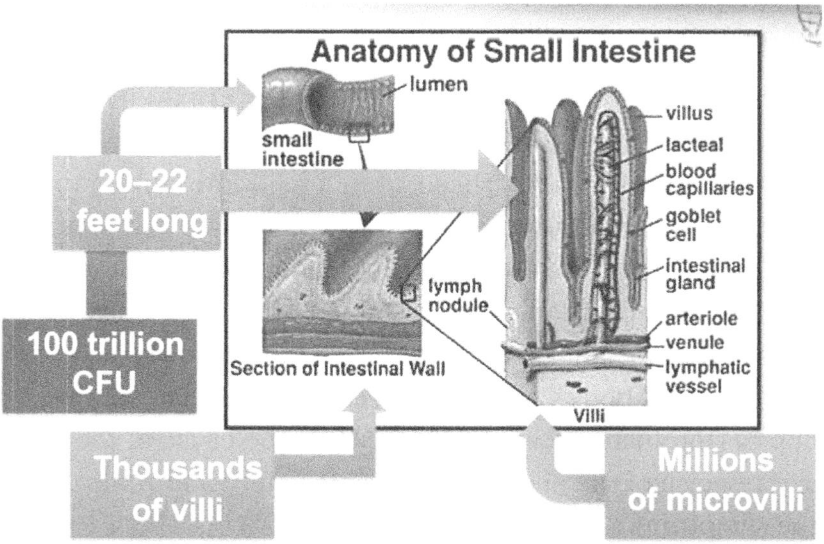

The only difference between the current medical view of the anatomy of the small intestines and the MMM interpretation are the 100 trillion CFU making up the MMM that protect and facilitate nutrient, waste, and microcontaminant flow through the intestines.

I consider the primary intelligence and function of the intestines resides in the software (the MMM), rather than the hardware (the anatomy).

CONCLUSIONS

Thus, allopathic medicine, which focuses more on body parts, cannot envision the value of the MMM. The cause, symptoms, prevention, and treatment of other "autoimmune diseases" are similar to the "autoimmune diseases" of the gastrointestinal tract. We will address diseases of other organs and systems categorized as "autoimmune disease" in our future book.

A breach of the MMM exposed to the external environment causes a cascade of breaches in mmm and tissue in pathways throughout the body. These breaches allow environmental contaminants to enter the body and accumulate in one or more susceptible organs or systems. The body's natural immune and inflammatory reaction, when sustained over a significant period, is diagnosed as autoimmune disease. Allopathic medicine tries to treat the body's protective responses, because they are unpleasant. Instead, we should focus on the cause of the breach and removal of the microcontaminants before and while treating the symptoms.

With this knowledge, we have answered the question of "what causes autoimmune disease?" that continues to perturb physicians and scientists.

CHAPTER FIVE

LUNG HEALTH

In medicine, we encourage our patients to eat a health-promoting diet and consume sufficient water to stay hydrated. Yet, how often do we speak to our patients about proper breathing and oxygenation? We can live weeks without food, days without water, and moments without oxygen.

It seems evident that as clinicians, the focus on pulmonary health should be of significant priority, not merely ensuring a patient does not have bronchitis, pneumonia, chronic obstructive pulmonary disease (COPD), or asthma. Rather, promote that the lungs are optimally healthy to help ensure the delivery of maximum oxygen to hemoglobin seeking the O2 molecule to perfuse through 60,000 miles of blood vessels in an adult body.

Pulmonary Terrain

The skin and gastrointestinal tract are routine discussion points in the primary care setting, as patients often present with dermatological or GI ailments. As detectives, the clinician explores potential causative agents from an epidemiological perspective. Yet, unless they are presenting with allergic-driven asthma, how often do we as clinicians consider the lungs as a massive interface with the patient's environment?

As with all tissues, the lungs also need oxygen to sustain and nourish them, including the alveoli. It has been reported that the lungs require 5 percent of total body oxygen consumption.[1] Adult human lungs inhale 8,000 to 11,000 liters of air per day, including contaminants, microbes, and fungal elements. We suggest a broader appreciation of how the lungs are not merely taking in oxygen; rather, the pursuit of the sustenance of life comes with risk and a physiological burden.

The health of the individual in a crowded public environment will be susceptible to not only pathogen exposure but also microcontaminant exposure. Flyers are all too familiar with inhalation of jet fuel and fumes as we board and taxi on the runway. The question is entirely reasonable to ask, what affect does inhaling toxic fuels or smoke have on the micro-environment of the lungs, not only mucus production from irritation, but also direct impact on the "lung microbiome?" It is reported by the Environmental Protection Agency that particulate matter (PM) of 2.5 microns or smaller raises a significant risk of entering the bloodstream and embedding in the alveoli (air sacs) of the lungs.[2]

An increase in average daily PM10 (particles < 10 microns) has been associated with an increase in mortality of 1.0% for the same and the following days.[3]

"Lung pollution" with small particulate matter increases mucus production, contaminates the lung tissue, and with natural moisture and body temperature, can dramatically increase the "petri dish effect" of the pulmonary system. A petri dish of human microorganism is maintained at body temperature, moisture, and has a growth medium much as mucus serves.

Existence of the Lung Microbiome

There is no longer a question if the pulmonary system has a microbiome. Just as the GI tract, oral cavity, vagina, and virtually all tissues and organs of the body, including the brain have a unique microbiome, so too does the pulmonary system. To quote the peer-reviewed literature:

> "The healthy lung was long thought of as sterile, but recent advances using molecular sequencing approaches have detected bacteria at low levels. Healthy lung bacteria largely reflect communities present in the upper respiratory tract that enter the lung via microaspiration, which is balanced by mechanical and immune clearance and likely involves limited local replication."[4]

A term far overused in medicine is the concept of healthy. Being healthy for one individual may be significantly different than for another individual. Reductionism, even at the level of BMI (Body Mass Index), although a yardstick for identifying an unhealthy trajectory, fails to capture variances of individuality, including muscle mass density.

In the world of primary care, pulmonary, and ears, nose, and throat (ENT) medicine, the overgrowth of "normal flora" is an all too frequent presentation. It would be great to have absolutes in clinical practice, yet since these do not exist in the truest sense, there are reference ranges clinically correlated with signs and symptoms. In the case of the lung microbiome, the scientific literature aptly describes it as follows:

> **"The nature and dynamics of the lung microbiome, therefore, differ from those of ecological niches with robust self-sustaining microbial**

> communities. **Aberrant populations (dysbiosis) have been demonstrated in many pulmonary diseases not traditionally considered microbial in origin, and potential pathways of microbe-host crosstalk are emerging."[4]**

Be sure to understand what the reference range represents. In some cases, it represents the average of society, where the average person is overweight, sedentary, eats poorly, and is generally unhealthy. In other cases, the reference range represents what is considered a target range representing the healthiest range.

The following diagrams contrasts the lung's physiological and pathological microbiomes.[4]

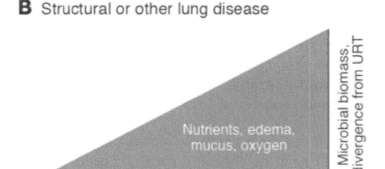

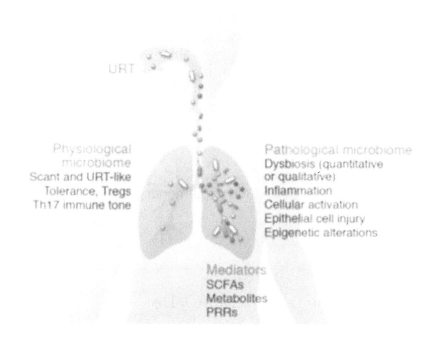

URT

Physiological
microbiome
Scant and URT-like
Tolerance, Tregs
Th17 immune tone

Pathological microbiome
Dysbiosis (quantitative
or qualitative)
Inflammation
Cellular activation
Epithelial cell injury
Epigenetic alterations

Mediators
SCFAs
Metabolites
PRRs

Exploring the Lung Microbiome

There are more questions than there are answers currently in the study of the lung microbiome. A dearth of research has been conducted in this burgeoning field. As clinicians and scientists, we seek more studies to appreciate pathophysiology and pulmonary health.

Suppose the lungs structurally and functionally fail to perform at peak levels. In that case, the entire body will suffer, including the microbiome, virome, and mycobiome. Furthermore, the balance between aerobic and anaerobic "biome" communities is in a constant state of changing equilibrium, potentially hindered by suboptimal oxygenation. Stated another way, "eubiosis" vs. "dysbiosis" is the proverbial Yin/Yang of any micro-ecosystem throughout the body. Oxygenation and deoxygenation are vital parameters for this ongoing attempt to maintain health-promoting homeostasis.

Lower oxygen concentrations are expected to be followed by increased levels of CO_2 (carbon dioxide), whose natural effect within the body is to acidify. Conditions that can most contribute to respiratory acidosis include:

- Asthma
- COPD (chronic obstructive pulmonary disease)
- Pneumonia
- Sleep Apnea
- Obesity
- Amyotrophic Lateral Sclerosis (ALS)
- Guillain-Barre Syndrome
- Restrictive Respiratory Diseases

Typically, the kidneys will offset respiratory acidosis with bicarbonate production (HCO_3). Yet, the body's acidity may increase with either primary kidney disease or secondary kidney function due to sustained hypoxia. Indeed, this change can also contribute to shifts in microbiomes throughout the body.

Metabolic Acidosis	Metabolic Alkalosis
Not reabsorting enough HCO3	Reabsorbing excess HCO3
Respiratory compensates by blowing off excess CO2	Respiratory compensates by retaining CO2

Clinical Practice and Pulmonary Considerations

In clinical practice over the last 30 years, Dr. Meletis has seen suffering from idiopathic pulmonary fibrosis, cystic fibrosis, COPD, chronic asthmatic changes in pulmonary function, and lung cancer impact his patients. With the epiphany of the existence of the lung microbiome, how does our therapeutic approach change?

Currently, it is postulated that the upper respiratory tract (URT) inoculum migrates in a diminishing gradient to the lower respiratory tract. Firmicutes and Bacteroidetes are the most common phyla, while Prevotella, Streptococcus, and Veillonella are the most common genera.[5, 6]

There is nearly identical composition of two adjacent communities, high microbial biomass (URT) and diminished microbial communities (LRT) (lung), suggesting that the lung microbiota is derived passively from the URT through microaspiration, which occurs even in healthy individuals.[7]

Yet, hematological sources of microbial changes within the lung microbiome have been documented. Lung infection from hematogenous sources arises from bacteremia and fungemia. Lung seeding with *Tropheryma whipplei*, typically considered a gut bacteria, is seen in asymptomatic people with HIV infection.[6]

Idiopathic Pulmonary Fibrosis

Idiopathic pulmonary fibrosis (IPF), a type of idiopathic interstitial pneumonia, is a chronic, debilitating lung disorder that results in a progressive worsening of lung capacity over time. It is characterized by scarring (fibrosis) and inflammation. The course of the disease can progress in varying ways, with some individuals undergoing periods of relative stability. In contrast, others experience a steady reduction in lung function or periods of acute exacerbation. Rarely, some patients may remain symptom-free for two to three years after diagnosis.[9]

In the United States, using narrow definitions, the prevalence is 14 to 27.9 cases of the disease per 100,000 population. Using a broader definition, the prevalence is 42.7 to 63 cases per 100,000 population.[10] IPF is slightly more common in males than females with a medium age of onset of 66 years.[11] Symptoms include shortness of breath and a cough, leading to marked declines in health-related quality of life. The survival rate is approximately two to five years.[10]

Conventional treatment for IPF usually includes corticosteroids or immunosuppressants, but this therapy does not markedly improve the survival of patients with IPF.[3] Balancing the benefits versus adverse effects of standard pharmaceutical therapies such as nintedanib, etanercept, warfarin (which is generally contraindicated), Gleevec, and bosentan is a very real clinical challenge.[12]

Studies report that IPF patients have higher bacterial load than healthy people. Both total bacterial burden and specific taxa (*Streptococcus and Staphylococcus*) are associated with more rapid disease progression. (Bacterial burden refers to harmful bacteria rather than bacterial balance called for in microbial mucosal milieu [MMM] theory.)   This raises the questions of causation of the imbalance and how best to alter the micro-terrain and microbial diversity to improve outcomes.[8]

Cystic Fibrosis

Cystic fibrosis is a genetic disease involving chronic inflammation and oxidative stress impacting the respiratory and digestive systems primarily. Cystic fibrosis is the most common life-shortening autosomal recessive disorder, affecting 30,000 people in the US and 70,000 globally.[14,15,7] Although 75 percent of people with the disease are diagnosed by age 2,[15] Dr. Meletis recently had a 12-year-old boy in his clinical practice diagnosed that was quite athletically active whose sole presentation was frequent congestion and phlegm particularly in the morning. This reminds us as clinicians to test patients with unique presentations.

A mutation in the cystic fibrosis transmembrane conductance regulator (CFTR) gene, leading to expression of impaired Cl- ion transport proteins in epithelial cells, is responsible for the development of cystic fibrosis.[14] This mutation results in insufficient hydration in the lungs and colon, leading to build up of viscous mucus on epithelial surfaces.[14,16] This accumulation of mucus leads to increased risk of infection in this group of individuals. Specifically, the lungs of cystic fibrosis patients are usually predisposed to colonization with *Pseudomonas aeruginosa* resistant to eradication by the immune system and medications.[17] The bacteria in the lungs of the cystic fibrosis patients often develops a biofilm to shield the microorganisms from host defenses and antibacterial drugs.[17] This biofilm combined with higher lung mucus viscosity and persistence in cystic fibrosis patients inhibits the effectiveness of antibiotics.[17]

Airway inflammation plays an important role in poor clinical outcomes in cystic fibrosis patients.[18] Inflammation markers are higher in the sputum of people with cystic fibrosis while anti-inflammatory markers are decreased.[19,20] Impaired fatty acid metabolism, including low omega-3 linoleic acid and docosahexaenoic acid (DHA) levels, have been observed in patients with cystic fibrosis.[21] Human and animal studies indicate that impaired fatty acid metabolism in cystic fibrosis patients may be associated with greater inflammation via an elevation in prostaglandin synthesis.[22]

Dysbiosis of the gut microbiota is another contributing factor in cystic fibrosis. We will discuss this and its relationship to MMM theory in more detail later in the chapter.

Asthma

Asthma is a chronic respiratory disease characterized by bronchial airway inflammation leading to increased generation of mucus and hyper-responsiveness of the airway to asthma triggers. Symptoms of asthma include wheezing, coughing, and shortness of breath. According to the Centers for Disease Control and Prevention, 18.4 million adults (7.6%) in the US have asthma.[23]

Genetic, allergic, environmental, infectious, emotional, and nutritional factors play a role in health of the airway MMM, where inflammation is posited to be the result of damage to the MMM, allowing environmental microcontaminants to breach the endothelial barrier of the airway. Whereas, researchers in 2001 proclaimed the cause of this inflammation to be an abnormal or poorly regulated CD4+ T-cell immune response.[24] Then a cascade of T-helper 2 (Th2) immune cells generates proteins known as cytokines, including interleukin-4 (IL-4), IL-5, IL-6, IL-9, IL-10, and IL-13. These cytokines enhance the growth, differentiation, and recruitment of mast cells, basophils, eosinophils, and B-cells. Each of these cells plays an essential role in humoral immunity, inflammation, and allergic response.

Chronic Obstructive Pulmonary Disease

Chronic obstructive pulmonary disease (COPD) is comprised of two conditions: emphysema and/or chronic bronchitis. Chronic infections are common in COPD patients, who have heightened inflammatory responses and a progressive reduction in respiratory function. Chronic cough, respiratory secretions, progressive difficult or labored breathing and fibrosis are all hallmarks of COPD. Nearly 15.7 million people in the US (6.4%) have COPD, although half of adults with low pulmonary function are unaware they have COPD so the actual number of people who have the disease may be higher.[25]

The primary cause of COPD is chronic exposure to cigarette smoke, and the risk of disease is correlated to the number of cigarettes smoked daily.[26] However, other contributing factors to the disease include high exposure to dust laden with toxins, contact with chemicals, and mutations in the α1-antitrypsin gene.[27,28]

Here we consider the impact of the microbial mucosal milieu relative to the microbial diversity in COPD. In a cross-sectional study of 72 COPD patients, airflow limitation correlated with increased relative abundance in sputum of *Pseudomonas* and decreased *Treponema*.[29] A study of 101 COPD patients found greater disease severity with increased Haemophilus and diminished *Prevotella* and *Veillonella*.[30]

Aeration (oxygenation of the LRT) may likely play a significant role in disease management as microbial profiles appear to be associated with bronchodilator responsiveness and peak expiratory flow rate in the SPIROMICS cohort.[31] Albeit a possible oversimplification, the concept of the MMM as the maintenance of the structural and functional integrity of the localized tissues is much like a well-regulated housing community with a good neighborhood watch. This is noted with the findings that lower microbial diversity of LRT is correlated with decreased lung function and frequency of acute exacerbation.[32]

Other Risk Factors for Development and Exacerbation of Lung Disorders

In addition to the risk factors mentioned above, there are several important contributors to the development or worsening of lung diseases.

Viral and Bacterial Infections

An association exists between infections with certain viruses and lung diseases, especially Idiopathic pulmonary fibrosis (IPF) and asthma. Studies using lung samples have established a possible association between the hepatitis C (HCV) family of viruses and IPF, acute exacerbations of IPF, or patients at risk for familial IPF, indicating these viruses may be involved in the development and/or worsening of IPF.[29] In one of those studies, HCV antibodies were present in 28% of patients with IPF compared with only 3.6% of controls.[30] In another study, researchers found a greater incidence of IPF at 10 and 20 years after HCV infection compared with hepatitis B virus patients.[31] Other researchers observed a greater prevalence of HCV in many forms of lung disease, indicating the association may not be limited to IPF.[36]

Scientists have also found the presence of herpes simplex virus (HSV-1) in bronchoalveolar lavage fluid and lung tissue biopsy from patients with IPF and nonspecific idiopathic interstitial pneumonia.[37] Epstein-Barr virus (EBV), which belongs to the herpes virus family, is also common in patients with IPF and may be involved in the development of pulmonary hypertension in these patients. [38-41]

Other viruses are implicated in the development or exacerbation of IPF. There is a high prevalence of the Torque-Teno (Transfusion-Transmitted) virus (TTV) in patients with IPF.[42] Furthermore, in one study, the three-year survival rate of patients with IPF who were infected with TTV was markedly lower.[42] The same trial also found higher TTV levels in patients with IPF who develop lung cancer compared to patients who did not develop cancer.[42] Additionally, TTV was the most common virus in a group of individuals with IPF suffering from acute exacerbation.[43] Scientists have also observed this virus in people with lung cancer and acute lung injury.[33]

Viral infections acquired early in life are also triggers for the development of asthma. A newly discovered virus family known as *Anelloviridae* are contracted in childhood and replicate continuously without causing any symptoms.[44] This virus modifies the innate and adaptive immune systems and plays a role in the development of asthma.[44]

Asthma may be associated with other types of viral infections including EBV[33] and adenovirus.[46-47]

Bacterial infections may also play a role in lung diseases. Interestingly, reports have identified *Chlamydia pneumoniae* infection as a trigger for the development of asthma and improvement in asthma occurred after antibiotics eradicated the bacteria.[48] *Chlamydia* infections may also worsen smoking-associated inflammation in COPD patients.[48] Another study in adults found that higher levels of *Chlamydia* antibodies correlated with greater asthma severity.[49]

Pseudomonas aeruginosa is another bacterial infection implicated in lung disease, specifically cystic fibrosis. Individuals with cystic fibrosis are vulnerable to P. *aeruginosa* infections of the lungs, and these infections are often resistant to clearance by the immune system and antibiotics.[17]

Gastroesophageal Reflux Disease

Gastroesophageal reflux disease (GERD) is characterized by reflux and regurgitation leading to symptoms such as heartburn, pain in the upper abdomen, difficulty swallowing, and aerodigestive symptoms including asthma, chronic cough, or recurrent pneumonia. GERD often occurs together with IPF and may play a role in progression and worsening of the disease.[50] Some evidence suggests that treatment of GERD leads to lower IPF-related mortality but not overall mortality.[50] **Researchers have also observed an increased incidence of GERD in asthma patients,[51] although it has not been firmly established whether these two disorders simply occur together, whether GERD causes asthma, or whether asthma causes GERD.[24] It is estimated that 75% of asthma patients have GERD symptoms, 80% have abnormal acid reflux, 60% have a hiatal hernia, and 40% have esophageal erosions or ulcerations.[51]**

Comorbidities are highly supportive of MMM theory. It is postulated that it is typical for a breach in the MMM in one organ or system to be highly correlated with a general state of dysbiosis of the MMM throughout the body. Adjacent MMM dysbiosis throughout the body are highly likely to impact one another or be affected by the microcontaminants that create a weakness in the local or adjacent MMM.

Increased bronchoconstriction occurs with esophageal acid infusion.[24] In a human study, this bronchoconstriction was eliminated after antacid symptom treatment.[52] The mechanism of action linking GERD to asthma may involve the vagus nerve creating a reflex from the irritated esophagus to the lungs, leading to bronchoconstriction. This is an interpretation of symptomatic association, rather than an appreciation of the MMM theory identified cause.[24] Another symptomatic rather than causal explanation is that gastric acid from the esophagus may seep into the lungs, causing injury, irritation, and increased mucus production.[24] This provides further insight into the potential symptoms arising from a weakened MMM in the stomach, esophagus, and lungs, where gastric secretions or hydrochloric acid is sloshing around damaging connecting tissues and organs rather than being contained by a healthy MMM, which may help protect the function of the lower esophageal sphincter.

There is some indication, as observed by Dr. Jonathan Wright, that asthma patients have reduced gastric acid output, which results in impaired protein digestion and nutrient absorption as well as increased food allergies.[24] MMM theory provides an alternative explanation.

Mouth, Ear, Nose, and Throat (M-ENT) probiotics plus colostrum is an MMM theory approach to avoiding and treating GERD. Supporting the integrity of the gastroesophageal MMM provides support and remediation of the MMM, minimizing and reducing inflammation and symptoms of GERD.

Gut Microbiota Affects Bronchial Function

An imbalance (dysbiosis) in the gut microbiota—the community of microbes residing in the intestinal tract—is associated with airway diseases such as cystic fibrosis and asthma. In cystic fibrosis, abnormal intestinal mucosa is associated with alterations in gut microbiota.[53] Patients with cystic fibrosis have a reduced overall bacterial abundance and lower species diversity compared with healthy people.[53] Researchers conducted one study of 43 individuals with cystic fibrosis and 69 controls without the disorder.[54] Although the greatest differences in diversity of the intestinal microbiota occurred between cystic fibrosis patients and healthy controls, alterations in the gut microbiota were also observed between individuals with cystic fibrosis when divided into groups based upon different parameters including the percent predicted FEV1 (a measurement of lung dysfunction) and the amount of intravenous antibiotic courses received in the previous year. Patients with cystic fibrosis who had severe lung impairment had markedly lower gut microbiota diversity compared with patients who had mild or moderate impairment. Additionally, a greater number of IV antibiotic courses was significantly associated with lower diversity of the gut microbiota. **Each of these comorbidities support MMM theory, the need for a healthy MMM, diversity of bacteria in the microbiome, and the unseen impact of environmental microcontaminants, especially antibiotics with a delivery mechanism as effective as IV, on the microbiota.**

There is also a relationship between gut microbiota and asthma. Infants given antibiotics have an altered gut microbiota and immune development and an increased risk of childhood asthma.[55] Likewise, in another study, similar associations were found for maternal antibiotic use before and after pregnancy. This indicated the correlation is either not directly causal or it's not specific to pregnancy.[55] This provides further evidence of the relationship of the gut MMM and comorbidities, where the child's microbiota is affected by the strongest anti-MMM treatment – antibiotics – whether dispensed to the child or to the pregnant or lactating mother. Furthermore, researchers have observed a difference in the gut microbiota profile of people with asthma compared with healthy controls,[56] further supporting comorbidity impacts of a dysbiotic MMM.

In mice with a predisposition to develop allergic airway diseases, oral administration of the live probiotic *Bifidobacterium adolescentis* ATCC 15703 alleviated allergic airway inflammation and decreased levels of eosinophils in the airway, hallmarks of allergic asthma.[57] In humans, supplementation with the probiotic L. *reuterii* was effective in reducing bronchial inflammation in children with well-controlled asthma.[58]

Another study evaluated the effects of supplementation with the prebiotic Bimuno-galactooligosaccharide (B-GOS) on exercise-induced bronchoconstriction and airway inflammation.[59] Ten adults with asthma and bronchoconstriction caused by hyperpnea (increased depth and rate of breathing) and eight healthy controls randomly received either 5.5 grams/day of B-GOS or a placebo for three weeks separated by a two-week washout period. The prebiotic intervention resulted in reduced airway hyper-responsiveness along with reductions in markers of airway inflammation.

Air Pollution and Environmental Exposures

Epidemiological evidence indicates there is a significant association between air pollution and the development and worsening of asthma and COPD. The primary components of pollution responsible are ozone (O3) and nitrogen dioxide (NO2), as well as particulate matter (PM) derived from car exhaust and industry.[9,60] Diesel exhaust particulate (DEP) can bind proteins and may act as a carrier of allergens, allowing them to penetrate deep into the respiratory tract.[9,60] Furthermore, acute flare ups and worsening of idiopathic pulmonary fibrosis correlate with exposure to O3, NO2, and particulate matter.[61] In addition, chronic exposure to air pollution might actually cause the development of Idiopathic pulmonary fibrosis (IPF).[61]

Indoor pollution including secondhand cigarette smoke and emissions from wood-burning stoves can also exacerbate asthma symptoms.[24] Secondhand smoke up-regulates the Th2 immune response in animal studies.[62] Exposure to cigarette smoke is also responsible for most cases of COPD.[63] Gas appliances can increase the level of nitrogen dioxide breathed in, impairing lung function.[24] Off gassing of volatile organic compounds (VOCs) and formaldehyde emitted from paints, adhesives, furniture, carpet, and building materials are also associated with an increased risk of asthma attacks.[24]

Airborne environmental contaminants often trigger asthma. My brother has asthma, likely related to higher levels of smog where he lives in Los Angeles. I was diagnosed with asthma after moving into my new house and having the contractor replaster, sand, and repaint the ceilings and walls due to drywall screw pops while we were living there. The contractor's standard of clean is "broom clean," meaning that not only do they circulate the settled dust when sweeping, but they leave a cloud of particulate matter as a result of "cleaning." When your HVAC ducting is "broom clean," your HVAC system basically becomes a circulatory system for environmental contaminants in your home. If you have HEPA filters installed, the particulates are caught at the point of the filters.

Your sinuses and lungs are much like HEPA filters. They capture tiny particulate matter, such as dust, pollen, other allergens, viruses, beneficial and harmful airborne bacteria, mold spores, paint fumes, and much more. Your lungs are particularly good at capturing all these environmental microcontaminants. What happens to all these environmental microcontaminants is dependent on the health of your bronchial MMM. Do these airborne microcontaminants enter your bloodstream, along with oxygen, or are they caught, degraded by beneficial bacteria in your MMM, and flushed via mucus to your stomach where they are further degraded and eliminated from your body?

When HVAC ducting is not properly installed, such as too severe bends in flexible ducting, condensation forms where airflow is disrupted at these bends, eventually followed by mold growth. Molds are serious environmental contaminants and do not belong in your HVAC system. In our new house, due to an intermittent water leak in the drain from our washing machine, which was not located for four months and happened to be directly above our HVAC system, the entire HVAC system, including ducting, became a toxic mold generation and circulatory system. Luckily, the temperature was moderate, and the HVAC system was not used much during the first four months after construction was completed and we moved into the new house. For the next year, the system was shut down. At the same time, the contractor and insurance companies fought over responsibility until I finally had the walls, ceiling and flooring ripped apart, and the HVAC units cleaned and discovered that the ducting was very poorly installed. Ducting was mostly replaced – Just no heat or A/C for the first year in our new home.

A robust respiratory MMM will protect and reduce the chances of irritating or toxic particulates entering the epithelial layer of your alveoli. See the next section and final chapter for a discussion about my asthma recovery after removing the precipitating factors – mold and dust – and supporting my respiratory MMM with detoxing probiotics.

Environmental exposure is also linked to IPF. A meta-analysis found that smoking at any time throughout life or exposure to agriculture/farming, livestock, wood dust, metal dust, and stone/sand were each considered significant risk factors for IPF.[35]

Critically Important Realization

In the field of medicine, we all must avoid *a priori* thinking and conceptualization. Each individual arrives at their unique health presentation via an individual journey. Though we know common pathophysiological processes, epigenetic factors must be considered to best explore this burgeoning field of the MMM. How did an individual's journey from *in utero* to the moment they present to the clinical setting create their own cellular and microbial trajectory. Do we look at an individual using a CPAP/BiPAP machine blowing positive pressure from the URT to the LRT as an individual at a unique risk of pulmonary disease? The answer seems to be yes, as they are altering their microecology with increased airflow that brings changes in humidity, and quantity of environmental contaminants.

It is also essential to look beyond bacterial diversity and explore the potential role of the lung mycobiome and virome. A significant challenge is the collection of unadulterated sampling from the LRT and the need for a more advanced testing methodology. What we do know is that relative to the mycobiome, "*Ascomycota and Basidiomycota* are the most commonly identified taxa, followed by the genera *Candida*, *Saccharomyces*, *Penicillium*, *Cladosporium*, and *Fusarium*." [64]

Natural Support for Lung Conditions

MMM Theory posits that supporting the microbial mucosal milieu in the lungs, sinuses, blood, and gut will decrease the entry of environmental contaminants, thus reducing the body's inflammatory and other protective mechanisms.

A robust respiratory MMM will reduce the risk of irritating or toxic particulates entering your alveoli and being carried throughout your body. However, there is a tipping point when even the most robust MMM will be overwhelmed with environmental microcontaminants.

Specific bacteria involved in detoxification may assist with the degradation and removal of a whole host of environmental microcontaminants, including BPA, perchlorate from jet fuel, pesticides, heavy metals, gluten, and sodium nitrate. Read more about these detox probiotics and how to support your MMM in Chapter 9.

Nutritional supplement discussion relative to lung condition is addressed in this chapter because oxygenation of all our tissues to create and sustain ecology for the microbial mucosal milieu to exist is oxygen dependent. Indeed, in the hierarchy of absolute necessity, we can live weeks without food, days without water, yet mere moments without air. Several nutritional and lifestyle options exist for patients with pulmonary concerns. Here are some suggestions based on both clinical practice and research.

Idiopathic Pulmonary Fibrosis. Animal studies have reported on the promising effects of several botanicals. In a rat model, rosemary extract, which contains rosmarinic and carnosic acids, reduced and cured pulmonary fibrosis even when it was administered after fibrosis occurred.[64] Similar results were achieved with rosemary extract in other animal studies.[65,66] Green tea is another botanical that has demonstrated anti-fibrotic activity in animal studies. In one of those studies, a rat model of pulmonary fibrosis, green tea extract reduced oxidative stress and suppressed endothelin-1 expression, a mediator of pulmonary fibrosis.[67] In another rodent model of pulmonary fibrosis, a combination of green tea extract and curcumin exhibited powerful, synergistic anti-inflammatory effects.[68]

Gingko biloba and carnitine were also studied in rats exposed to a substance that causes pulmonary fibrosis.[69] Researchers induced pulmonary fibrosis in the animals then administered Ginkgo or carnitine. Ginkgo decreased the collagen content in the lungs of the rats and reduced inflammation and oxidative stress. Carnitine did not reduce the collagen content but did lower oxidative stress and inflammation.

Additionally, promising results were achieved using *Rhodiola rosea L.* in a rat model of pulmonary fibrosis.[70] Rhodiola protected against fibrotic lung damage through its anti-inflammatory, antioxidant, and anti-fibrotic actions.

Furthermore, a combination of the botanicals *Astragali Radix, Angelicae Sinensis Radix, Paeoniae Radix Alba, Pheretima, Chuanxiong Rhizoma, Carthami Flos,* and *Persicae Semen* (known as a Buyang Huanwu decoction) alleviated pulmonary fibrosis of rats by improving lung tissue morphology and reducing levels of serum collagen types I and III.[71]

Human studies of dietary supplements and IPF have focused on the use of N-acetylcysteine (NAC). A meta-analysis found that although NAC did not have a beneficial effect on changes in forced vital capacity, changes in predicted carbon monoxide diffusing capacity, rates of adverse events, or death rates, NAC did significantly improve decreases in percentage of predicted vital capacity and six minute walking test distance.[72] Inhalation of NAC is a promising route of administration as noted in a study where patients with early stage IPF experienced enhanced forced vital capacity after exposed to NAC in an aerosol form.[73]

Cystic Fibrosis. In addition to supplementation with probiotics, as noted earlier in this chapter, there is also justification for support with other nutraceuticals in patients with cystic fibrosis. An imbalance in omega-6/omega-3 polyunsaturated fatty acids is common in cystic fibrosis (CF) patients.[74] Consequently, researchers have explored the effects of omega-3 fatty acid supplementation in these individuals. One randomized, placebo-controlled study found that compared to the previous year, cystic fibrosis patients given omega-3 fatty acids experienced a decline in pulmonary exacerbations at 12 months.[75] In addition, the subjects receiving the omega-3 fatty acids took antibiotics for a shorter period of time (26.5 days compared with 60 days in participants not receiving the fatty acids.)

NAC is another nutraceutical studied in patients with cystic fibrosis. When combined in an inhaled form together with an aerosol form of an antibiotic drug, it has synergistic effects against P. aeruginosa infections in this group of patients.[17] NAC is known for its ability to break down mucus. Therefore, combining it with the drug, enhanced the ability of the antibiotic to diffuse into the mucus, compared to when the drug was used alone.

There's also indication that vitamin A may play a role in the health of cystic fibrosis patients. After excluding subjects with acute pulmonary exacerbations, researchers found that cystic fibrosis patients with a moderately high retinol level (up to 110 µg/dL) had the best respiratory function without any signs of toxicity.[76]

Asthma. Since oxygen radicals play a prominent role in the development of asthma, antioxidant supplementation is important. In one study, levels of antioxidant vitamins C and E were low in the lung lining fluid of individuals with asthma, despite normal or increased plasma concentrations of the vitamins.[77] Furthermore, vitamins E and C may be able to prevent air pollution damage in patients with asthma. Four randomized, controlled trials found that vitamin E combined with vitamin C protected against bronchoconstriction caused by ozone in people with and without asthma.[78-81] Furthermore, the gamma-tocopherol isoform of vitamin E suppressed markers of inflammation in subjects with asthma and reduced acute airway response.[82]

Vitamin D is another nutrient of interest to asthmatics. Although not all studies have found an association between vitamin D and asthma, enough evidence exists to warrant its use. Three population-based studies demonstrated a correlation between lower serum vitamin D concentrations and severe asthma exacerbations or core measures of exacerbations such as hospitalizations.[83-85] For example, one of these studies observed that vitamin D insufficiency or deficiency in Puerto Rican children is linked to increased likelihood of having had one or more severe asthma exacerbations in the previous year.[83]

Other nutrients that may be important for individuals with asthma include pyridoxine (vitamin B6), magnesium, and omega-3 fatty acids.[86-88]

One botanical showing promise in supporting asthma patients is Boswellia serrata, which suppresses the formation of leukotrienes, inflammatory metabolites of arachidonic acid. One double-blind, placebo-controlled trial investigated the effects of 300 mg Boswellia extract three times daily for six weeks in 40 subjects with asthma.[89] Symptoms such as difficulty breathing, number of attacks, and wheezing improved in 70% of the participants given Boswellia compared to only 27% of the placebo group. Measurements of lung function also improved in the patients given Boswellia, and eosinophilia was reduced.

The connection between GERD and asthma and the finding that stomach acid is low in asthmatics indicates there may be justification for use of *Boswellia* extract.[24] Moreover, in some people with asthma, aspirin or other non-steroidal anti-inflammatory drugs (NSAIDs) can trigger an attack, so avoiding this class of drugs is important.[24] By blocking the cyclooxygenase enzyme, NSAIDs lead to production of leukotrienes, which in turn promote inflammation and bronchial constriction.[24]

Dehydration may also play a role in asthma symptoms.[90]

Chronic Obstructive Pulmonary Disease.

Dietary supplements can offer support to COPD patients. Carotenoids and vitamins D and E help suppress lung injury after pollution exposure.[91] Furthermore, nitric oxide (NO) modulates lung function, and low serum NO concentrations are associated with COPD severity.[92] This indicates that NO-balancing supplements such as L-citrulline and beetroot juice may be beneficial.

Additionally, NAC may be beneficial in COPD. In patients with COPD who were at high risk for exacerbations, a randomized, placebo-controlled trial showed that 600 mg twice per day of NAC was associated with a reduction in exacerbations and increased the time to the first exacerbation.[93] In another trial, Chinese patients with moderate-to-severe COPD given 600 mg of NAC twice daily for a year experienced a reduced number of exacerbations, especially in patients with moderate disease severity.[94, 95]

Conclusion

Our lungs are vulnerable to an onslaught of toxins, including cigarette smoke and indoor and outdoor pollution. Lung disorders can seriously affect the quality of life and in the case of idiopathic pulmonary fibrosis, significantly increase mortality. Supporting your pulmonary MMM, as we discuss in Chapter 9, will reduce the body's burden, degrade, and remove airborne toxins. Incorporating specific nutraceuticals into the regimens of patients with pulmonary concerns and in some cases implementing lifestyle solutions can help sustain lung health.

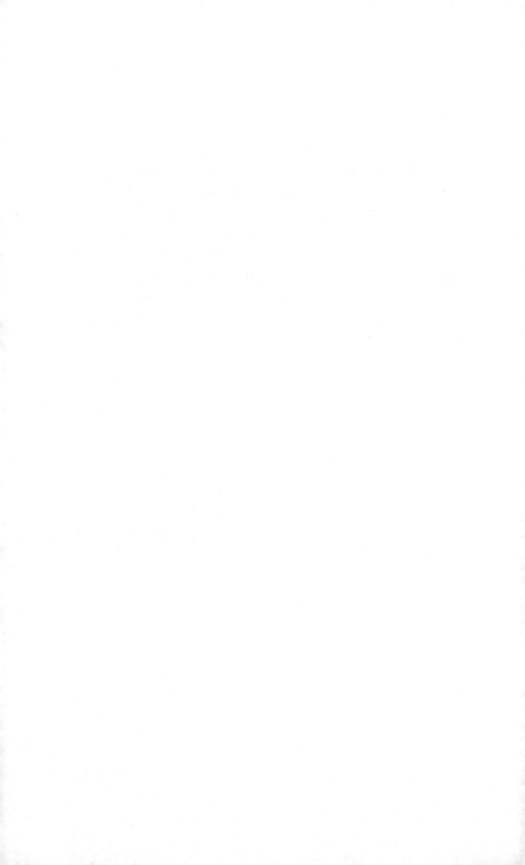

CHAPTER SIX

BRAIN, BBB & NEUROLOGICAL MMM

To organize and process new experiences and sensory data, human nature often defaults to comparisons. This observational predisposition can be both helpful and a limiting hindrance, particularly regarding innovation and scientific exploration. With discussion of the microbiomes beyond the gastrointestinal tract, we must approach investigation with the open mind of an explorer observing and pondering a never-before-seen discovery.

The GI microbiome has been exhaustively studied relative to other microbiomes throughout the body. Our scientific approach must not only be through the lens of the GI microbiome; in addition, we must appreciate each ecosystem (microbiome, mycobiome, and virome) of a given tissue or system in its own light. To think of the skin, lungs, cardiovascular, or other tissue and organ microbiomes ONLY as they compare to the uniqueness of the gastrointestinal tract would be like looking at a ruby, emerald, or sapphire only as if it were a lesser form of diamond. The perspective of the Microbial Mucosal Milieu (MMM), a new and expansive paradigm and lens, assists us in appreciating the intricate microbiota network within and between regions of the body.

Under normal homeostasis in a healthy individual, the neurovasculature confers meaningful brain protection. However, in states of inflammation, integrity of the BBB can and does become compromised. We live in a time where inflammation secondary to a westernized diet and lifestyle has experienced a significant uptick. This prevalent state of being has fueled the concept of Inflamm-Aging that was coined in scientific literature in 2000.

Let's take a moment to ponder what is healthy and by whose definition. Would we say in North America that 20 percent of the population is robustly healthy defined as disease free, optimally nourished and rested, and with a healthy mucosal membrane defense? Whatever the number, optimal health seems elusive, as we have seen rises in autism, Alzheimer's disease, cancer, and cardiovascular disease over the last decades. Further confounding the definition is the concept among functional medicine providers of subclinical disease states. A classic example is the thyroid patient that presents with normal thyroid hormone lab indices, TSH, Free T4, Free T3, and antibodies. Albeit often marginally normal, they present with classical signs and symptoms that respond to low-dose thyroid replacement. So, are these individuals healthy before or after treatment?

The concept and clinical discussion of the presence of a leaky gut impacting and causing a leaky brain was recently a foreign concept in clinical practice. Most clinicians were taught and indoctrinated that the BBB is the ultimate fortification against pathogens and nefarious agents that would affect the human central nervous system.

We have known for decades that cerebral spinal fluid can be measured via procedures such as a spinal tap (lumbar puncture), and infectious agents can be quantified, thus guiding therapeutic interventions. A presentation of infectious encephalitis is then treated, and if symptoms abate, the general trend assumes the patient has resolved the infection. How often does a lumbar puncture occur in a newly recovered patient that has been successfully treated? With the risk of introducing infectious agents, this is not a proposition that is taken lightly. How do we know that the brain has returned to normal homeostasis, or might there be a residual altered brain microbiome, virome, and mycobiome? In recent years, advances in sample collection that are sufficiently clean, meaning they are devoid of potential contaminants introduced during extraction and testing, and the development of greater sensitivity of 16S RNA gene amplification and in situ staining technology to test remote low-density microbial burden tissues have become available.

There are three primary ways to define the gut-brain connection – cross-talk, blood-brain barrier (BBB) disruption, and studying microbes in the brain.

Cross-talk between gut microbiota plays a fundamental role in modulating many gut-brain axis-related diseases, including gastrointestinal disorders and psychological diagnoses. Similarly, gut hormones also play pleiotropic and important roles in maintaining health, and are key signals involved in gut-brain axis. Peer-reviewed literature suggests that cross-talk disruptions between the GI tract and central nervous system (CNS) may contribute to the pathogenesis of various neurodevelopmental disorders. Conditions that once were believed to fall into either gastroenterology or neurology are now viewed as sharing a more intricate and complex pathophysiology such as IBS, autism, anxiety, attention-deficit hyperactivity disorder (ADHD), and obesity.[1]

BBB disruption may arise when allostatic load exceeds the

body's ability to acutely or chronically adapt. There are many disease states, and physiological stressors can alter the functional integrity of the BBB.[2,3] Both hypoxia and inflammatory processes change the BBB's permeability properties and the pathophysiology of CNS diseases, which can also contribute to altered therapeutic strategy and efficacy.[4]

There is clear and intriguing evidence for the presence of microbes in the human brain. This has been noted in cases of brain injury observed in HIV/AIDS accompanied by microbial brain infiltration.[5] Only time will reveal all the pathways in which the brain's microbiome is populated including blood, lymph, neuronally and beyond.

Bacterial Case in Point

It is reported that upwards of 10 percent of the healthy populace has Neisseria meningitides in their nasal passages. N. meningitides in susceptible individuals, can enter the bloodstream via type IV pili on bacterial surfaces, passing endothelial cells, allowing entrance into the meninges of the brain thus breaching the blood-brain barrier.[6]

Celiac Case in Point

Often referred to as gluten ataxia, individuals with overt Celiac disease can manifest with CNS symptoms. They may also display dermatological presentations as dermatitis herpetiformis. The CNS, dermatological, and other manifestations of a GI condition point to not only the importance of looking at disease states beyond their immediate locale or presentation epicenter, but also the genesis and ripple effect throughout the body. In the spirit of this book's discussion of the MMM and the proposed interconnectivity and communication between previously believed isolated micro-ecologies, for every action and reaction in one part of the body, there can be broad and consequential effects throughout multiple MMM barriers and conduits. As an analogy, a tsunami may be triggered on the other side of the Pacific Ocean yet come ashore thousands of miles away with local inhabitants (in this case, distant tissues and cells) not having any sense of how, when, or why pathophysiological and biochemical changes in their immediate terrain were triggered.

A closer look at celiac disease is suggested to better set the tone and embrace whole-body medicine. It is well established that celiac disease has a highly variable (inter- and intra-individual) presentation that can alter multi-organ systems, including the CNS. Some of these symptoms may be due to altered nutritional status. The gluten-consuming patient will have routinely experienced atrophied villi limiting nutrient absorption and conceivably disrupting brush border enzyme production.

Extra-intestinal celiac complications have been reported to include cortical hyper-excitability and neurological and motor cortex involvement.[7] Some individuals with celiac disease will also experience altered cognitive processes and symptoms, cerebellar ataxia, neuropathy, seizure, headache, and neuropsychiatric presentations.[8] As with other CNS-presenting conditions, inflammation appears to be the critical marker in altered blood-brain barrier integrity. It should be noted that non-celiac gluten sensitivity has also manifested with neurological and neuropsychiatric presentation.[9]

MMM Theory explores the question of a breach exclusively in the gut microbiome versus a cascade of breaches beginning with an external microbiome, such as the gut, sinus, or skin microbiome, and also presenting as a breach in the blood and BBB microbiome. Comorbidities are supportive of this cascade of damage caused by environmental microcontaminants. One example of these comorbidities is demonstrated by 60 percent of children diagnosed on the spectrum having GI issues and 40 percent of these patients having sinus or allergy issues.

Among the Many Mechanisms of Altered BBB

Thus far, we have discussed a few examples that establish that the BBB has vulnerabilities. Yet there are indeed circumstances that lead to altered BBB clinical presentations that may or may not be directly created by an altered brain microbiome or, at the very least, an altered brain terrain.

Attributed to both Socrates and Plato, the following quote is still pertinent in the 21st century and the field of research and medicine: **"I am the wisest man alive, for I know one thing, and that is that I know nothing."**

This chapter is not a treatise on all the mechanisms that may disrupt the BBB, but rather an appreciation that it does become disrupted. As with all other microbiome alterations, MMM theory postulates that related BBB microbiome changes may, and likely will, occur elsewhere in the body. Thus, comorbidities are expected. The global MMM impact on the CNS begs the question: when a patient presents to their PCP or specialist with an atypical presentation and is told it is all in their head, is that indeed a greater truth than we expected?

There are likely many pathophysiological mechanisms at play that can alter the BBB in isolation or in concert, including overt IgE-driven food and environmental allergies, IgG or IgA-driven food, or aeroallergen sensitivity, plus potential mycotoxin exposure. There is also emerging attention being given to glycotoxins linked to inflammation.[10] Indeed the inflammasome – comprised mainly of the cytokines interleukin (IL)-8, pro-inflammatory cytokines tumor necrosis factor (TNF)-α, and interferon (IFN)-γ – likely play a role in the inflammatory process leading to localized changes in tight junction proteins.[4]

Cross-Talk Between the Brain and GI Microbiome

MMM theory posits that microbiota from one part of the body may directly influence or inoculate another region. Additionally, the MMM is a confluence of more than microbes and byproducts of metabolism locally and globally of the host and the symbiotic non-self.

Communication from the gut microbiome to the central nervous system (CNS) occurs via many mechanisms. These include microbial-derived intermediates, short-chain fatty acids (SCFAs), secondary bile acids (2BAs), and tryptophan metabolites.[11,12] The abundance of both immunological and neurological activity that arises from the GI tract speaks volumes to supporting the long-held premise, postulated by Hippocrates in 400 BCE, "All disease begins in the gut." Though likely overstated to a degree, the lack of a healthy GI tract alters everything from nutrient absorption and immune reactivity to neurotransmitter balance (locally and globally). It increases the risk of invading toxic microbes impacting local and distant tissues and organs.

Neurological Connectivity

Cranial nerve 10, the vagus nerve, connects our CNS with the GI tract. Indeed, the vagal nerve lives up to its nickname, the vagabond nerve, as it wanders throughout the GI viscera and communicates at a postulated 80 percent afferent (sensory) to the brain as to the state of affairs within the GI tract directly affecting digestion. The right and left vagal nerves comprise 75 percent of parasympathetic nerve fibers and have an integral role in heart rhythm.

Vagal Nerve Involvement:

- Digestion
- Heart rate
- Blood pressure
- Respiration (breathing)
- Immune system responses
- Mood
- Speech
- Mucus and saliva production
- Urine output

Enterochromaffin cells in the GI tract store serotonin (neurotransmitter) and are integral to vagal neuron sensing that occurs within the gut. Nutrient digestion, eubiosis, and dysbiosis impact enteroendocrine and enterochromaffin cell functions. These factors result in reactivity within the mucosal membrane immune system, triggering release of intermediates across the intestinal barrier that enter systemic circulation and can even cross the blood-brain barrier.[13,14]

It is important to note that microbial signals communicate via neural pathways involving vagal and spinal afferents.[15,16]

Glymphatics and Beyond

Microglia account for 10 to 15 percent of all brain cells and are distributed throughout the CNS. They are resident macrophage cells and act first and foremost as a form of active immune defense in the central nervous system (CNS).

Microglial cells are involved with antigen presentation, phagocytosis, and modulating inflammation.[17] Microglia provide surveillance of the CNS environment while directly communicating with neurons, astrocytes, and vasculature.[18] Microbial-derived SCFAs promote microglial maturity and proper functioning, thus showing interwoven dependence of the body's microbiome and brain sustenance.[19]

First described in 2012, glymphatics have been demonstrated to provide far greater passage of materials in and out of the CNS than previously thought. The CNS was previously believed to be isolated. Yet, how could it survive without delivery of nutrients and removal of waste?

> **"The glymphatic system is a recently discovered macroscopic waste clearance system that utilizes a unique system of perivascular tunnels, formed by astroglial cells, to promote efficient elimination of soluble proteins and metabolites from the central nervous system. Besides waste elimination, the glymphatic system also facilitates**

> **brain-wide distribution of several compounds, including glucose, lipids, amino acids, growth factors, and neuromodulators. Intriguingly, the glymphatic system functions mainly during sleep and is largely disengaged during wakefulness."** [20]

Again scientists show that once steadfast beliefs regarding the function and what might be construed as limitations of the body and brain are now being expanded. Researchers also found that the glymphatic system delivers nutrients to the CNS, allowing it to be a potential delivery mechanism of environmental microcontaminants. Indeed, as clinicians and researchers, it is time to fully embrace the *Star Trek* saying, **"Where no man has gone before."**

Microbiome, Virome, and Beyond

When examining a patient's clinical manifestation of either peripheral or central neuropathogenic presentation, we must examine the individual's wellness and burdens. We must not just look at the anatomical brain as we were taught in Biology 101, but rather the complexity of the neuro-network and the potential of microcontaminants, as noted throughout this chapter. Indeed there is a GI-Brain axis, a microbiome, mycobiome, and invariably a significant likelihood of a brain virome even in a non-symptomatic individual.

Peer-reviewed literature is growing in both depth and breadth relative to the influence of the gut and whole body microbiome. They influence neuropsychiatric conditions, including depression and anxiety, autism spectrum disorder (ASD), schizophrenia, Parkinson's (PD), and Alzheimer's disease (AD).[21-24]

When pondering CNS and peripheral neuropathic presentations, the presence of a brain or localized virome-driven dysfunction must be part of the differential diagnosis. Researchers have identified a relatively high prevalence of qualitative "brain virome" existing as the herpes virus in human brain samples. The herpes genomic sequences of HSV-1 were seen in 28-100 percent of samples[25,26] or HSV-6 in 2-70 percent.[27,28]

Thomas Edison has been quoted, ***"The Chief Function of the Body is to Carry the Brain Around."*** A deeper examination of this quote speaks to how the brain needs the body and brain co-existence is intricately interwoven and dependent. To think that the body's global health and, in turn, the MMM does not impact the brain and vice versa is yesteryear's thought processes that merely serve to limit more rapid advances in all fields of medicine.

CHAPTER SEVEN

CIRCULATION AND LYMPHATICS

As we explore the presence of the Microbial Mucosal Milieu (MMM) within the blood circulatory system and lymphatics, we must re-evaluate what is considered "healthy" or "friend vs. foe" relative to microbes. When, where, how, and why does a tipping point manifest in an individual or organism so that a disease state is identified, quantified, and thus considered for treatment?

An adult's vast circulatory system traverses the body's far reaches via some 60,000 miles of blood vessels. 60,000 miles is impressive itself, but imagine this represents a surface area of at least 2 (Π) R times that length, believed to total about 3,000 square meters, greater than half a football field. This entire surface area needs to facilitate protection, ingress, and egress of nutrients, waste, and all kinds of signaling molecules.

The oldest understood function of oxygenated and nutrient-rich blood is to sustain structure and function. The microbial mucosal milieu serves an integral role in arterial blood delivery of nutrients, oxygen, and beneficial bacteria to mitochondria and cells. The MMM in venous blood returning to the liver and heart acts as a conduit for waste, microbes, and microcontaminants.

New research shows that blood flowing through our body may not be sterile as once thought. Additionally, all blood from the gastrointestinal tract flows to the liver via the portal vein. The moment we eat and consume bacteria, fungi, viruses, combined with endogenous resident living organisms within our GI tract we are inoculating the bloodstream. This is further amplified for those with excess intestinal permeability, commonly known as leaky gut.

A healthy GI tract is selectively permeable, allowing for the absorption of vitamins, minerals, nutrients, and a portioned amount of microbial and foreign antigen exposure to sustain a competent and mature immune defense system. It is when EXCESS contaminants in any form permeate into circulation that signs and symptoms of altered physiological functioning present as a "disease state." So, the term "leaky gut" and all its current representations need to be clarified to represent excessive permeability rather than normal permeability. A similar case could be made for the lymphatic system.

There is growing evidence that there is indeed a blood microbiome, albeit the concept is not broadly appreciated or embraced. Overt blood-borne bacterial infections, bacteremia, have long been diagnosed and treated, as the pathogenesis and clinical presentation have hit the threshold of diagnostic and clinical appreciation. Yet as clinicians and researchers, we must stay humbled by the lack of knowledge and technological advancements.

Recalling back to the proverbial dark ages of medical science, it took Louis Pasteur's experiments to disprove the theory of "Spontaneous Generation," in which living organisms can be derived from non-living matter. Yet such was the thought within the medical community. As I have shared with colleagues over the years, we can pride ourselves in the tremendous strides science has made; we have increased diagnostics, advanced therapeutics, and a much deeper appreciation of the nuances of human disease. Yet, in a mere five years, new research will challenge even the brightest minds and long-held concepts. For a moment, think of the advances in your area of expertise and how it has changed how you would have treated a patient 10 years ago if you knew what you know now.

Thanks to the introduction of Next Generation Sequencing (NGS), identifying and quantifying our unique "microbial selves" via whole metagenome shotgun sequencing (WMGS) allows us to explore the presence of non-human genomics in the various structures of the body.

This chapter focuses on the dissemination of microbial communities throughout the body via circulatory and lymphatic systems. Beyond the intestinal microbiome, scientific literature supports the presence of microbiomes in the lungs, skin, eyes, mouth, placenta, genital-urinary tracts, and elsewhere.[2,3,4]

Among domesticated birds and mammals, a blood-microbiome has been noted, including healthy young cats and chickens with osteomyelitis.[.] A compelling demonstration of the fluidity and interconnectivity of the MMM has been demonstrated in mice when an acute instillation of LPS into their lungs changed the composition seen in the gut, blood, and lung microbiota.

There are three important articles in the early 2000s that advanced human blood microbiome research. In 2001, a small study demonstrated the presence of bacterial DNA in "healthy" individuals' blood via qPCR that included rRNA-specific fluorescent probes and 16S rRNA gene-specific primers. The study identified bacterial taxa belonging to five divisions and seven phylogenetic groups.

Research in 2002 showed the presence of pleomorphic bacteria in asymptomatic individuals. The findings confirmed the presence of bacterial DNA in the blood of "healthy" individuals. The techniques used were transmission electron microscopy (TEM), dark-field microscopy (DFM), fluorescence in situ hybridization (FISH), and the sequencing of PCR-amplified 16S rRNA and gyrB genes.

In 2008, another study confirmed the presence of bacterial 16S rRNA genes in healthy blood.

Still a Lack of Consensus

As with all medical paradigm changes, some researchers are still looking to validate the presence of microbes in healthy individuals. Thus, the discussion will continue. However, the concept of microbes and other non-self organisms in the blood of "healthy" individuals seems to be a certainty, though clinical mindset often changes at a glacial pace. The National Institutes of Health reports that new research takes an average of 17 years to reach clinical practice. Three studies by Balas and Bohen, Grant, and Wratschko all estimate an average lag time of 17 years using different evaluation criteria. Imagine how dogmatic and out of date are some doctors who are at the tail end of the average range.[29]

With recognition of the presence of microbes in blood, the ripple effect in the medical model will be far-reaching. Currently, blood used for transfusions is routinely tested for an array of viruses, HIV, Hepatitis, etc., yet might a broad bacterial spectrum actually be protective? This concern was captured in a 2016 article and its dogmatic conclusion:

"We demonstrate that a diversified microbiome exists in healthy blood. This microbiome has most likely an important physiologic role and could be implicated in certain transfusion-transmitted bacterial infections. In this regard, the amount of 16S bacterial DNA or the microbiome profile could be monitored to improve the safety of the blood supply."

As a disruptive hypothesis, MMM Theory posits that there exists a healthy and beneficial microbiome in blood and vasculature. If so, the perspective may become to support transfusion of blood along with blood MMM as a protective agent against "certain bacterial infections."

Dental Health and Heart Disease

Study participants with poor oral hygiene (never/rarely brushed their teeth) experience an increased risk of cardiovascular disease. It has long been appreciated that dental procedures can lead to bacteremia, hence the use of antibiotic prophylaxis as a standard of care. These findings help connect the dots that bacteria and antibiotics are disseminated via the blood. Furthermore, antibiotics such as amoxicillin significantly impact bacteremia after a single tooth extraction. Yet a more significant question was raised by authors in the journal *Circulation*.

"... given the greater frequency for oral hygiene, tooth brushing may be a greater threat for individuals at risk for infective endocarditis."

Dormant Bacteria

It has been postulated that some micro-organisms in blood may indeed be dormant (non-culturable). Non-culturability may be partly due to insufficient technological advances, a desire for a silver bullet culture rather than culturing a complex community of bacteria, and bacteria residing in the intracellular space of red blood cells. These findings are clinically relevant as these microbial sources can fuel inflammatory, non-inflammatory, and potentially immunological reactivity secondary to molecular mimicry.

> "A number of recent, sequence-based and ultramicroscopic studies have uncovered an authentic blood microbiome in a number of non-communicable diseases. The chief origin of these microbes is the gut microbiome (especially when it shifts composition to a pathogenic state, known as 'dysbiosis')." [14]

> "Another source is microbes translocated from the oral cavity. 'Dysbiosis' is also used to describe translocation of cells into blood or other tissues. *To avoid ambiguity, we here use the term 'atopobiosis' for microbes that appear in places other than their normal location.* Atopobiosis may contribute to the dynamics of a variety of inflammatory diseases." [14]

MMM Theory suggests the paradigm may need to shift. Rather than assuming and looking for dormant bacteria that are potentially displaced and harmful, one should be open to a vast community of non-culturable bacteria that are symbiotic, beneficial, and may balance any harmful bacteria.

MMM Theory posits that the MMM undergoes constant adaptation to the changing host and external environment while continuously seeking homeostasis. Is the old paradigm of culturing a single bacterium still meaningful, or does that reflect silver bullet dogma that may not be appropriate for achieving homeostasis in a community of bacteria? In the new paradigm, how will an historical snapshot of a few culturable bacteria be interpreted to provide value?

The MMM Is Not Limited to Bacteria

The term microbiome is often used in the medical literature to reflect bacterial colonization and presence. However, the clinical picture is incomplete without including the mycobiome (fungal) and virome (viral).

Technological advancements and methodology relative to low abundance within blood samples have limited quantification of *Archaea* and lower eukaryotes (such as fungi). It's critical to delineate that low does NOT mean absent. A 2014 study demonstrated a 0.01 percent presence of circulating archaeal DNA in "healthy" individual blood samples. There is growing evidence circa 2018 that the presence of fungi in "non-diseased" individuals is highly likely.

The authors of the 2018 study share their conclusions:

> **"Here we demonstrated rich biodiversity of naturally occurring bacterial and fungal blood microbiota in healthy individuals."** [16]

> **"For the first time we identify rich fungiome in the blood."** [16]

> "This work brings evidence, that the resident blood microbiota in healthy individuals should be considered non-pathogenic and a normal feature of healthy blood."

The clinical relevance did not escape the authors as they presented their conclusion:

> "Furthermore, we anticipate our resuscitation strategy and sequencing approach to be a model for studying numerous chronic diseases, such as obesity, diabetes, cardiac failure, liver diseases, hematologic disorders, neurodegenerative diseases and chronic infections, like latent tuberculosis. Beyond cataloguing species of the blood environment, the blood microbiome field will focus on defining mechanisms underpinning interactions between microbes and host, mechanisms influencing initiation and progression of diseases with a view towards personalization of patient's diagnosis and treatment." [16]

Virome

Testing for past, present, and reactivated viral infections in the clinical setting is relatively routine. Yet, the question from a public health perspective and societal construct makes the conversation on viral load and prevalence in non-symptomatic individuals a hotbed of potential controversy and therapeutic consideration.

As noted throughout this chapter and others, the concept of "healthy" or "non-diseased" is somewhat arbitrary. What truly is healthy or non-diseased?

In a study published in 2017, 19 viral taxa were noted in 42% of overtly non-diseased individuals.[17] Other studies have confirmed the presence of anelloviruses, *Herpesviridae*, rhabdovirus, and *Poxiviridae*.[18,19,20]

Lymphatic System and the MMM

As discussed in the brain/central nervous system chapter, we once believed that the brain was sterile, much like dogma has held for sterility of the bladder, blood, and countless other tissues and organs. Indeed "immunoprivileged" body sites, if any, are diminishing. And it is not just our blood vessels that serve as conduits for cross-talk between various microbiomes.

Researchers have identified lymphatic vessels that transport immune cells and fluid from the brain's cerebrospinal fluid (CSF) and cervical lymph nodes. Study authors shared the following important insights.

> **"We show that dural lymphatic vessels absorb CSF from the adjacent subarachnoid space and brain interstitial fluid (ISF) via the glymphatic system."[21]**

> **"Overall, these data indicated that lymphatic vessels are present in the dura mater of the CNS and drain out of the skull via the foramina of the**

base of the skull alongside arteries, veins, and cranial nerves." [21]

Suppose one was to be so bold as to realize that both blood vessels and the gut now appear to be conduits of bacterial, fungal, and viral translocation. The GI tract is permeable by nature; thus the concept of a leaky gut is a misnomer if used to designate a pathological state. Rather, "leaky gut" is more correctly "hyper" permeability that within susceptible individuals presents with a cascade-triggering event at the immunological and inflammatory level. We believe it can be argued that a "healthy" populace has an acceptable level of "leaky gut" that should be considered normal. "Hyper leaky gut," while not identified as such, has been the focus in clinical and research settings. We propose that immune competence requires a degree of immune tolerance that arises upon modest exposure (i.e., your immune system develops as it is exposed to a low level of antigens). If your gut allowed "no leakage," your immune system would not develop. Current "leaky gut" discussions do not differentiate between passage of nutrients and waste and passage of harmful microcontaminants. The dialog needs to be clarified to explain this complexity. MMM Theory proposes this discussion.

The concept of compartmentalization of truly "closed systems" seems to be an artificial construct that time has passed. After centuries of studying the human body, we only have a grasp of its complexities. As seen in this 2016 article in Nature, we are still discovering new physical structures within the body.

> **"In searching for T-cell gateways into and out of the meninges, *we discovered functional lymphatic vessels lining the dural sinuses.* These structures express all the molecular hallmarks of lymphatic**

endothelial cells, are able to carry both fluid and immune cells from the cerebrospinal fluid and are connected to the deep cervical lymph nodes." [22]

"The discovery of the central nervous system lymphatic system may call for a reassessment of basic assumptions in neuroimmunology and sheds new light on the etiology of neuroinflammatory and neurodegenerative diseases associated with immune system dysfunction." [22]

The role of the lymphatic system and inflammatory bowel disease also clearly demonstrates that microbiota within the mesentery lymph varies and that a microbiota presence is quantifiable. These findings were shared in the *Journal of Crohn's and Colitis* in 2019.

> "This study confirms that there are distinct differences between Crohn's disease (CD) and ulcerative colitis (UC) mesenteric lymph node [MLN] microbiomes. Such microbial differences could aid in the diagnosis of Crohn's disease or ulcerative colitis, particularly in cases of indeterminate colitis at time of resection, or help explain their mechanisms of development and progression."[23]

Maintaining tissue integrity and controlled permeability while clinically looking to sustain a healthy or less pathophysiological structural integrity is essential. The authors speak to their further findings.

> "Mechanistically, the gut microbiota reportedly restricts translocation of pathogenic bacteria to the MLN. This may be compromised in CD but not

UC, because the MLN microbiota of CD patients displays an overabundance of *Proteobacteria* [known to contain numerous pathogenic species]. Likewise, the clearance of harmful bacteria from MLNs could also be reduced." [23]

The Source of Our Inoculum

If we were born sterile, with a non-existent MMM, where would we receive our inoculum? New scientific literature abounds with how our inoculum is sourced. Our inoculation begins *in utero* before birth via vertical transmission. There is a prenatal blood microbiome based on the isolation of bacterial DNA from the umbilical cord of C-section-delivered healthy babies. Vaginal delivery and breastfeeding also contribute to the creation of the newborn's MMM and neuro-immune development.

Several other sources throughout our maturation contribute to our MMM development and potential disruption. It has been postulated that the development (to some degree) of conditions such as liver cirrhosis, blood disorders, diabetes, and cardiovascular disease may arise from the translocation of harmful bacteria from the gastrointestinal tract, skin, and oral cavity.[26,27,28]

In MMM Theory, we postulate that the translocation of beneficial bacteria are related to lack of development of conditions such as liver cirrhosis, blood disorders, diabetes, and cardiovascular disease.

Why is it called "leaky gut" when an environmental contaminant enters circulation via the gut, versus when a protein or beneficial bacteria enters the blood or glymphatic system from the gut? Is this leaky gut hypothesis not screaming for clarification such as MMM Theory?

The MMM in Clinical Context

For eons, humanity has co-existed with bacteria, viruses, and fungi; thus, it is not so much that some of the discoveries should be surprising or alarming per se. MMM theory raises the question of what is considered "normal, healthful, and pro-homeostatic."

The host organism (patient) has an ever-changing variable degree of susceptibility to acute and chronic disease, flares of these conditions, and the ability to regain homeostasis. Succumbing to an "unhealthy state" is impacted by various epigenetic risk factors and prior injury.

A proactive approach to a globally healthy MMM includes sustained health of all the individual microbiomes and, equally important, the cellular and tissue integrity of the tissues and organs throughout the body. Indeed, structure begets function, and function begets structure.

6 Steps for MMM Management

1. Whole body nourishment (micro and macro nutrients) along with phytonutrients, from a highly varied diet

2. Augment the microbiome of each smaller "mmm" community to sustain the global MMM

3. Nourish immune competence

4. Control microcontaminants that serve as disruptors of the MMM

5. Sustain the integrity of each of the individual microbiome communities to enhance inter-MMM communication and support

6. Adhere to a wellness regime that minimizes stress, supports optimal sleep, and lessens allostatic load

Each organ and tissue of the body "cross-pollinates" its unique MMM with near and distant individual MMM communities. In its entirety, it can be viewed as many smaller "mmm entities" that when viewed as a whole create the larger Microbial Mucosal Milieu that is essential to the co-existence of "us and them," a designation in and of itself which is archaic. **As we are them, and they are us! Indeed, WE ARE!!**

CHAPTER EIGHT

SKIN MICROBIOME

Skin is one of the largest human organs and communicates with the external environment in a bi-directional fashion via excretion (generally sweating), absorption, and touch as a means of bacterial translocation. The skin surface area is, on average, 30 m^2 (323 square feet) for an adult.[1] Something that seems so easy to calculate – the surface area of the skin – has been underestimated for decades. Initial calculations did not consider pores and hair follicles. Current calculations demonstrate that skin surface, literally visible for all of us to see, is indeed 10 times greater than previously believed. This new calculation takes into appreciation the surface area of the skin that is exposed to bacteria; thus the size of our dermal Microbial Mucosal Milieu (MMM) may be 10 times greater than thought, and larger than our gut MMM, but far smaller than our vascular MMM. It should give us all pause and appreciation for other closely held beliefs that may need to be further explored.

> "If one estimates the depth of an average human follicle to be 3 mm and the diameter of that tube is approximately 0.5 mm, then the surface area of a hair follicle is 3.14159 × 0.5 × 3 = 4.71 mm^2 or 4.71 × 10^{-6} m^2. The human body is estimated to have 5 × 10^6 follicles. Therefore, the surface area of the follicular surface could be approximated as 4.71 ×

$10^{-6} \times 5 \times 10^6 = 24$ m². Added to the 2 m² surface area estimate based on the exposed interfollicular epithelium and considering that other appendage structures like sweat and sebaceous glands also provide epithelial surfaces for microbes, the total skin surface area is at least 30 m². This is more than 10 times greater than the surface area commonly reported for the skin!"[1]

Different parts of the body have bio-diverse microbial communities that reside in systems and organs throughout the body. Interface of microorganisms helps sustain proper skin functioning, no different than any other microbiome located within the body, gastrointestinal tract, blood, bladder, lungs, etc.

Disrupting the skin microbiome and MMM can result in dysbiosis and manifest as part of the pathophysiological processes of dermatological conditions.

We have routinely been taught to judge a patient's health not just by the book but by its cover, yet the human body cover (the skin) can tell the observant clinician many a clue of the state of internal homeostasis.

Points of Consideration:

- Radiant glow (health from within)
- Pallor (anemia, malnourishment, sympathetic nervous system)
- Jaundiced (liver disease, hemolytic anemia, premature infant)

- "Green around the gills" (idiom of nauseated or ill)
- "Rosy complexion" to reflect a state of health

Average skin thickness is a mere 2 to 3 millimeters (about 1/10 of an inch). Yet, our very existence is dependent on these millions of cells for their protective role, thermoregulation, water conservation, noxious stimuli avoidance, and as a location of vitamin D synthesis.

An optimal dermatological microbiome is the foundation of the skin's immune system. Though there is a dearth of data on phages due to their low gradient biomass in skin samples, they serve an important role in sustaining function and composition of the microbiome.[2,3]

The microbiome of "healthy" skin comprises a complex diversity of bacteria, fungi, viruses, mites, phages, and archaea.[4,5] Thus giving us pause as clinicians about being allergic to dust mites. However, dust mite triggered immune reactivity is quite common and thus consuming crustacea such as shrimp, crab, lobster, etc. can further burden an already stressed immune system. In short, if one reacts to dust mites one is in a perpetual state of reactivity.

Diverse Body Ecology

Depending on the skin's moisture and environmental humidity, the quantitative abundance of bacteria varies, all other things being equal. In moist areas such as the axilla, nostrils, and groin, bacteria colony count routinely exceed 10^6 CFU/cm², whereas, in less moist areas, colony count is 10^3 to 10^4 CFU/cm².[6] Variance of bacterial abundance based on humidity and temperature raises the clinical question of whether dehydration, moisture changes associated with aging, indoor heating, and outdoor climate may alter the skin microbiome. It seems evident that certain dermatological conditions appear more prevalent in high-humidity regions of the world, such as fungal infections. Notably, the predominant component of the skin microbiome and MMM are bacteria with the following distribution.[7]

Human Skin Bacteria Classification

- Actinobacteria   52%
- Firmicutes   24%
- Proteobacteria   16%
- Bacteroidetes   6%

Creating and sustaining an appropriate terrain, a flourishing health-promoting skin microbiome, and MMM is essential. Thus, it is wise to control for deleterious variables that affect skin ecology and increase the risk of dysbiosis.

Select Factors that Affect Skin Ecology:

- Hydration
- Body and skin pH
- Blood sugar
- Exposure to "other" skin microbiomes (intimate

partners and family members), hand railings, doorknobs, gasoline nozzles, elevator buttons, sports and workout balls and equipment, etc. We call your awareness to things which are never cleaned.

- Utilization of various soaps (antibacterial vs. non-antibacterial)
- Chlorinated water bathing
- Hot tub, swimming pool, community gym
- Topical creams, lotions, shampoo (exposure to chemicals such as paraben and other noxious agents)
- Makeup, cologne
- Sunscreen

In clinical practice, we routinely meet patients on their dermatological journey, having been stuck in a catch-22 use of antibiotics (topical and/or oral), steroids (topical and/or oral), and, at times, even biological prescriptions. One of the most common prescriptions that Dr. Meletis has seen for his patients with atopic dermatitis (eczema) is the "prescribed bleach bath" by their dermatologist or allergist. The recommendation of immersing the body in dilute bleach speaks to a non-holistic approach to the MMM and microbiome. Bathing in bleach is akin to using a broad herbicide to kill weeds in the lawn, yet laying waste to the lawn and weeds alike.

There is no question that bleach (sodium hypochlorite) is an effective antimicrobial which is routinely used as part of backyard and public pool maintenance and cleaning. Tap water from municipalities is routinely treated with chlorine and chloramine, as stated on the EPA's website:[8]

Chloramines (also known as secondary disinfection) are disinfectants used to treat drinking water, and they:

- Are most commonly formed when ammonia is added to chlorine to treat drinking water.
- Provide longer-lasting disinfection as the water moves through pipes to consumers.

    According to the EPA, water that contains chloramines and meets EPA regulatory standards is safe to use for:

    Drinking

    Cooking

    Bathing

    Other household uses

As noted in the text box above, bathing water contains chloramines or has been chlorinated. In clinical practice, a dechlorinating filter for the shower or bathtub is vitally important in reestablishing and maintaining an optimized microbiome and

MMM. A person will also notice that their hair and skin are much softer after a shower or bath that contains no chlorine.

Re-Inoculation of the Skin MMM

Re-inoculation of the microbiome and the global MMM after a bleach bath, chlorine shower, or use of alcohol carriers in cosmetics must be approached with a broad and holistic view. As clinicians, there is a broad array of gastrointestinal, vaginal, oral, and skin probiotics that can be employed in the clinical setting. MMM theory suggests that all these endothelial body surfaces display similar, yet localized, functions. And all display similar, yet different, localized microbiome composition as described in Chapter 3 – Where is your MMM?

However, there are limitations to these approaches, as merely repopulating an unhealthy terrain does not resolve the underlying issue that leads to dysbiosis. Thus, a comprehensive protocol in manifesting a robust skin MMM includes:

1. Optimize body pH and nutritional status with a healthy, balanced diet, but not with alkaline water or acid reducing/blocking drugs

2. Proper hydration

3. Avoid excess hygiene with antimicrobials; avoid chlorine and chloramine exposure orally and topically

4. Focus on a healthier terrain for your global MMM (skin and beyond)

5. Ensure detoxification via skin, liver, GI, and kidneys (organs)

and that blood, lymph, mucus, urine, feces (pathways) are supported

Lay of the Land and Skin

Human skin is slightly acidic at a pH of approximately 5.6; however, physiological changes can change systemic and dermal pH. Epidermal skin turnover occurs about every 28 days, with the average adult exfoliating nearly a million or more cells per hour.[9] As we ponder the body-wide MMM and ways that our regional MMM (aka "mmm") auto-inoculate one another, it is interesting to note that about 10 percent of exfoliated skin contains bacteria that we invariably inhale (lung) and ingest (GI).[6,10]

The primary residents of the skin are bacterial commensals. However, it is more than just a numbers game, as the integrity and resilience of skin MMM arises from a balance of diversity within the dermal microbiome in the perpetual effort to avoid a dysbiotic state. There is indeed strength in numbers and a dynamically integrated community to confer immunological protection beyond skin deep.[11]

Common disease processes associated with altered skin microbiome include acne, dandruff, and atopic dermatitis.[12-14] Both dandruff and seborrheic dermatitis have been associated with an overgrowth of *Malassezia* yeast, a resident microbiota of healthy skin, and likewise, psoriatic lesions commonly experience excess *Malassezia spp.* and *Streptococcus species*.[15,16]

Gender – More than Skin Deep (The Microgenderome)

Individual skin microbiome is as diverse as unique human beings. Factors that impact our skin MMM include but are not limited to health status, age, sex, personal hygiene, geography, environment, and the health of individual microbiomes within the body.

Sex-specific differences relative to the dermal microbiome and potential clinical therapeutics are worth consideration. The following simplified comparative listings are merely generalized observations and individual differences within XX, XY, and chromosomal variants at both the genotype and phenotypical levels.

Other factors at play include differences in sex hormones between

---

Sex-Specific Microbiome [6,17-19]

Males tend to have:

- Thicker skin, more body hair and sebaceous glands

- Lower microbial diversity

Females tend to have:

- Thinner skin, less body hair, and fewer sebaceous glands
- Higher microbial diversity

sexes and among a given chromosomal presentation. They can vary widely in youth, puberty, menopause, and andropause (male menopause).[20] Likewise, anatomy appears to matter when it comes to microbial diversity, as the surface of women's hands show greater diversity than those of men. Women's hands had more Lactobacilli spp and Enterobacter spp. in contrast to men that had more *Cutibacterium* and *Corynebacterium*.[6,21]

Handing Off Microbial Diversity to the MMM

The scientific literature strongly suggests influence of sex, hormonal maturation, and differences in structural genitalia anatomy and resultant variances in the microbiome. The local microbiome of our hands alone begs the question of cross-talk, the cross-cultural interplay between various regional microbiomes, and ultimately, sophistication and maturation of our collective MMM. Indeed, our microbiome(s) and the microgenderome play an integral role in immune competence as well.[22]

Auto-Inoculation from one microbiome to another can strengthen immune competence unless a highly virulent pathogen is at play. In a 2015 study the following findings were observed in medical students regarding "hand-to-face" touching frequency, including touching mucous membranes:

> "On average, each of the 26 observed students touched their face 23 times per hour. Of all face touches, 44% (1,024/2,346) involved contact with a mucous membrane, whereas 56% (1,322/2,346) of contacts involved nonmucosal areas. Of mucous membrane touches observed, 36% (372) involved the mouth, 31% (318) involved the nose, 27% (273)

involved the eyes, and 6% (61) were a combination
of these regions."[23]

In short, welcome to the cross-inoculation of various regional
microbiomes from other regional microbiomes. Hand from the
bathroom, hand to the cell phone, hand to the door handle, then
hand to eye, nose, throat, or feeding oneself. How many uniquely
defined microbiomes were just inoculated?

Auto-inoculation from the skin to mucous membranes, inhaling
and ingesting skin and other particles, or breathing communal
lung air in a closed space; we are a collective of MMMs, and
we have been for millennia and have survived. Indeed, there is
strength in numbers, diversity, and clearly strength in a mature
and competent immune system.

Thus, MMM Theory characterizes a new circulatory system that
has not yet been called out in scientific literature – touch – as a
circulatory system.

International Skin Microbiome

It appears that inhabitants of our planet may have unique skin
microbiomes. The modern world is becoming ever smaller with
international travel, immigration, emigration, and international
cuisine; it is time to apply a global lens to dermatological
presentations and health. Thus greater diversity is expected.
However, skin microbiome (mmm) interface with total body
MMM promotes rapid or dramatic shift without time to adapt or
evolve. This abrupt evolutionary change can trigger individual
immune dysfunction.

In the proverbial melting pot of humanity, what is the impact on humanity's MMM, individually and collectively, as we inhale, ingest, touch and otherwise inoculate one another?

Here are sample characteristics from scientific literature relative to regional inhabitants.

> East Asian individuals have a unique microbiome compared to Caucasians and Hispanics.[17]

> The quantity of *Cutibacterium* on the scalp and armpits of males in Africa and Latin America are lower than Caucasian, African–American, East Asian, and South Asian males.

Another study demonstrated uniqueness of microbiota on the hands of women from America and Tanzania. It revealed the possible influence of environment on microbiota on the body's surface.[24] These generalized findings may be attributable to hygiene practices, use of soaps, essential oils and water purity, diet, humidity and even type of clothing worn - breathable vs. layered, synthetic fibers vs. natural cotton, wool, hemp, etc.

Additional Factors Impact the Skin Microbiome and MMM

The use of cosmetics, UV exposure, chemical sunscreen, antibiotics, synthetic or petroleum-derived clothing, and several other factors impact the robust nature of the skin microbiome. A local professor of dermatology notes that psoriasis patients are often sensitive to black clothing dye, elastic, residual embedded herbicides, detergent, perfumes, and clothing softener residue, and more, which may each trigger a psoriatic reaction. She begins treatment by removing the precipitating factors.

It is routine practice in the Covid-Era to be very sanitary and "germ aware," yet in the process of targeting potential pathogens, we are also disrupting our friendly flora and the micro-environment in which bacteria flourish and protect us.[5]

Clinicians are familiar with UV radiation as a means of sanitizing and, at times, a therapeutic to treat various dermatological conditions. Indeed, many patients have noted resolution of skin ailments after a summertime of sunshine and fresh air. Whether intentional or not, by living inside and rarely being exposed to natural UV rays, or using sunscreens that block UV rays, impacts the MMM; or being a big outdoor person also influences the health of the MMM.

Antibiotics are a double-edged sword, as they assist the immune system in controlling "select bacteria." Yet, their reach is often far too broad, hence the term broad-spectrum antibiotics. We may seek to treat bronchitis or sinusitis yet inadvertently affect not just the GI tract but the skin and many other local microbial mucosal milieu. Here are some observations from recent scientific literature.

> With prolonged acne therapy, macrolides increased the number of C. acnes with decreased macrolide sensitivity. Research has demonstrated that erythromycin and azithromycin-resistant strains can range from 50 to 100%.[25,26]

Antibiotic Selection Can Impact the Microbiome Differently

> Oral minocycline decreased the skin microbiome colonies of Corynebacterium, Cutibacterium, Lactobacillus, Prevotella, and Porphyromonas.[27]

> Altering the microbiome comes at the risk of dysbiosis. Oral doxycycline had significant impact

on the following bacteria:[28]

- *C. acnes* decreased 1.96 fold
- *Snodgrassella alvi* decreased 3.85-fold
- *Cutibacterium granulosum* increased 4.46 fold

Likewise, Lymecycline, a tetracycline derivative, decreased the presence of *Cutibacterium* while it increased the number of *Corynebacterium*, *Micrococcus*, *Staphylococcus*, and *Streptococcus*.[25]

A point to ponder is antibiotic resistance in bacterial skin cultures. As we auto-inoculate the rest of our body's MMM, what impact do "altered" bacteria have on other microbiome communities?

It is important to note that whenever we apply anything to our skin, there will be one of three outcomes: improvement, neutrality, or detrimental impact on healthy biodiversity. An example of a positive influence would be the skin microbiome stimulating effect of hyaluronic acid precursor molecule N-acetylglucosamine.[14]

Pajama Therapy–Microbiome Transplant

Re-establishing a health-promoting skin microbiome once it has been disrupted is vitally important. In clinical practice, Dr. Meletis routinely utilizes "pajama therapy." The concept is simple. Dr. Meletis identifies a family member with good overall health and, most importantly, healthy skin. He will have the skin microbiome donor wear pajamas (their sleepwear) for between one and three nights, and then without washing the outfit, he will have the recipient wear the same sleepwear for a couple of nights. This process is repeated with a fresh set of sleepwear for two to four weeks to help re-establish a familiar/familial skin microbiome. Skin-microbiome transplant in various manners has been explored in the scientific literature.[29-32]

More than Skin Deep – The Dermatological MMM

To advance the field of medicine, both clinically and research-driven, we must move beyond thinking in terms of areas of specialty, subspecialty, and artificial boundaries of individual organs and body systems. The human body and its commensal microbiome are far more complex than our current technology allows us to appreciate. We all inherit "a train of thought," the prevailing wisdom of those who proceed us in our respective fields. Yet much like current knowledge dwarfs what was known just a few years ago, likewise, what we hold steadfast as an absolute may or may not withstand the test of time.

We know that the skin and its microbiome are essential in maintaining our well-ordered physiological processes. This includes the host's immune system function. Our skin and its MMM are part of a larger whole-body ecology. When we treat one part of the body more often than not, we treat other regions that initially seem remote and unrelated. As the tide rises, all ships rise; and the counterpoint, as the tide falls, so do all the ships.

CHAPTER NINE

DIET, LIFESTYLE, AND
SUPPLEMENT CONSIDERATIONS

Imagine for a moment walking in the shoes of your ancestors just 200 years ago. What did they eat? How did they wash and prepare their food? Did they have running water? How "clean" was the place your relatives were born and raised?

Or imagine walking in the "shoes" of your ancestral bacteria which evolved to become human mitochondria. The research supporting mitochondrial evolution is presented in Chapter 3 – Where is my MMM?

Don't get us wrong; there have been tremendous advances in hygiene, disease-free water and food, yet at what price has it come? The goal of this book is to raise awareness that there is still much to be appreciated about the complexity of our relationship with our microbial friends and foes. A global full body MMM exists and it communicates and is a conduit for regional microbiomes throughout the body. The MMM is an organ(ism) that is not contained by a single organ, tissue, or body region; it is a community or collective.

In our quest to eradicate disease-producing pathogens, we have harmed our friendly flora and their symbiotic impact on us. It is not practical or possible for current medical science to selectively target "bad" bacteria. Indeed are bad bacteria always bad, or are some only interpreted as bad actors when out of balance?

What follows are practical ways to bring some balance into our modern lives, provide a healthier life for your Microbial Mucosal Milieu, and thus directly improve health and disease trajectory. The evolving application of fecal transplants as a therapeutic intervention suggests a burgeoning appreciation of "Stool Pills or Enemas" as a treatment for C. difficile. Fecal transplants are also used off-label for anxiety, depression, autism, and more. How many years ago would a fecal/brain connection been considered heresy?

Certainly, there has been "better living through chemistry," (thank you DuPont) yet so has there been environmental and ecological damage that includes our human ecology or microbiome. Herbicides, pesticides, plasticizers, xeno-estrogens have impacted animals, our pollinators, and yes our MMM.

The following health and wellness considerations are presented to enlighten, empower, and re-establish what has been traded away over the course of the last 120 years or so.

We have established a primary root cause of diseases classified as "autoimmune disease," and diseases where inflammation is a symptom or perceived cause.

The overall approach to preventing and treating all these "diseases" is to support the microbial mucosal milieu (MMM), reduce environmental contaminants, then support natural tissue rebuilding and cellular energy:

1. Remove precipitating factors – those environmental toxins that damage the MMM, allowing microcontaminants to

enter and circulate through the body.

2. Support the MMM with diet, lifestyle, and supplements to restore its health and protective effect.

3. Remove/detoxify circulating and stable/lodged microcontaminants. Reducing the toxic burden lessens the need for the body's protective (chronic inflammatory) and isolating (in fat deposit) responses.

4. Provide support to calm the inflammatory cascade and the tissue damage that it causes.

5. Provide support for the restoration of mitochondria, cells, and tissue that were damaged by the body's protective mechanisms (inflammation, bleeding, diarrhea, coughing, fat deposition, etc.), which have been attacking these microcontaminants.

6. Reduce EMF exposure.

7. Provide ongoing maintenance support for the MMM because it will always be exposed to MMM-damaging toxins in our modern environment.

All of these considerations can be prioritized to:

a. Clean up your diet by minimizing packaged, processed, and fast food. Substitute with freshly prepared food. Leftovers count as freshly prepared food!

b. Minimize exposure to an environment that contains the toxins that we have identified in Chapter 2: You are Being Poisoned.

c. Take targeted detox probiotics to reduce microcontaminants in your body. Ask a naturopathic or other qualified Doctor about chelation and cleanses.

d. Increase variety in your diet and supplements to obtain the diversity of nutrients that your body needs to avoid episodic nutrient deficiencies that contribute to diseases of aging.[1] A sophisticated multivitamin is a fundamental way to cover your bases.

e. Supplement with a diversity of probiotics, naturally occurring in some foods, and with probiotic supplements that support your MMM.

f. Supplement with high-quality colostrum which complements and significantly increases the effect of probiotics.

g. Provide diet and supplements that support your mitochondria. These include CoQ10, PQQ, red spinach extract, L-Arginine, epicatechin, and supplements that boost your NAD+ availability.

h. Provide diet and supplements which support healing and tissue growth. These include amino acids in whey protein and colostrum.

i. Minimize EMF exposure.

j. Continue with pharmaceutical medications that your doctor may have prescribed to treat your symptoms. Talk with your doctor about reducing your pharmaceutical drugs as you restore your MMM and reduce your microcontaminant load, sometimes referred to as microcontaminant body burden.

Reduce and Protect Against Environmental Contamination

Living environment

One option is to live in a bubble. Given that is not practical for anyone, the next best is to spend more time in a cleaner environment. Outdoors is often cleaner than indoors. In the mountains, at the beach, and in the desert tend to be preferred locations. Even if it is just for a vacation, you're giving your body a breath of fresh air and time for your innate detox systems to catch up.

But be careful with short-term rentals in a tropical or humid climate. Some I have visited have had visible mold in the air conditioning units if you look closely. So, you're constantly circulating mold inside the home.

Next is to change out the cleaning chemicals in your home and office. Plant-based cleaners tend to be less harmful to your MMM because they do not use hydrocarbon derivatives.

Take care of a water leak immediately. This is a high potential source of mold.

Visible mold is often a marker for hidden mold. Mold clearance is generally not a do-it-yourself project. Catch it early to minimize clearance cost. For non-porous surfaces, white vinegar is a better mold cleaner than bleach, and much safer and more pleasant smelling.

Always open a window or use the exhaust fan in your bathroom when showering to clear moisture to prevent mold growth. If there are screens on the windows, clean them occasionally so they do not become a mold growth matrix.

Diet

Your diet means everything. In general:

Fresh food is better than packaged food.

Freshly prepared food is better than packaged prepared food.

Organic is better than non-organic.

Food grown without pesticides and herbicides are better than otherwise, even if they are not certified organic. A local farmers market is a great source of food, supporting your local community. Commercial crops used in packaged and prepared foods such as wheat, corn, soybeans, flax, and many others are generally grown with herbicides. Herbicides on the plant surface can be washed off. Herbicides that are absorbed by the plant from the soil, surface application, or water, become a part of the plant that you eat.

Frozen and refrigerated non-processed foods are generally better than canned and highly processed foods.

Watch out for antibiotics in food. Shredded cheese, whether from the grocery store or a fast-food outlet, almost always is packaged with antibiotics. Though, sometimes shredded cheese is packaged with microbial enzymes to kill mold. Enzymes are preferable to antibiotics in not damaging your MMM. The large surface area on shredded cheese will grow mold much faster than a brick of cheese, which you can shred when you want shredded cheese. Anything on the other ingredients list ending in *mycin is an antibiotic. Avoid foods that contain antibiotics added to reduce bacterial, mold, and mildew growth. These antibiotics damage your MMM.

Water

Never drink alkaline water. It neutralizes the ability of your stomach to protect you against harmful bacteria, mold, and viruses, whether you breathe them in, eat them, or drink them.

In the same way, acid-blocking prescription and over-the-counter drugs, such as proton pump inhibitors (PPIs) all have a short-term use recommendation, because they destroy your body's ability to protect you against harmful bacteria, mold, and viruses. Pharmaceutical companies and your doctors may not know why there are so many side effects of pharmaceutical drugs, but they are generally aware of the side effects. MMM Theory provides an explanation for some of these side effects.

Recall that mucus in your lungs clears your lungs of mold, harmful bacteria, allergens, particulates, and viruses. Mucus flows from your lungs and sinuses to your stomach where the highly acidic conditions are supposed to kill the microcontaminants. These microcontaminants will not die if you have neutralized your stomach acid with alkaline water or PPIs.

Don't drink or shower in chlorinated water. Chlorine is added to public water to kill bacteria in your water supply, but you don't want the chlorine to enter your body and kill the 90% beneficial bacteria in your GI tract, sinuses, lungs, and on your skin.

There are a number of water filter systems available for you.

They include whole house water filters (not necessarily for hard water, but to remove chlorine and chloramines).

Installing a whole house water filter will help minimize further copper pipe damage. Expect it will cost a few thousand dollars, but that is much less costly than one or more pinhole leaks and the ensuing mold remediation and rebuilding your walls, ceilings, floors and damaged furniture and storage that may be caused by a pinhole water leak and mold growth. Sorry for the news and yet something else to think about, but I have had too much experience with this, as it has caused damage to my home, my office, my furniture and electronics, and my health.

Other options for removing chlorine and chloramines, and other water-borne toxins include point of use filters. These include kitchen and shower water filters.

A good shower water filter is designed to remove chlorine and chloramines from hot water, and thus protect your lungs from a chlorine gas shower. Look for a shower filter that is labeled for use with hot water. They are available at most big box hardware/home centers.

The type of kitchen water filter I prefer is a reverse osmosis (RO) water filter. You will be amazed at the difference in the taste of your water. The health benefits for your MMM are substantial. Newer models of kitchen water filters cause the water to be alkaline. Avoid these at all cost. I'm not convinced that a simple water filter in a pitcher removes enough chlorine and chloramines to protect your health. But each step you take is beneficial and reduces the cumulative toxic body burden.

Just imagine if these chlorine and chloramine molecules can destroy metal (copper pipes), what type of damage they do to the beneficial bacteria that makes up your MMM and subsequently to your tissue. And yet, your public water provider uses these chemicals – their intent is that the water does not contain harmful bacteria, but while killing the harmful bacteria, they're also killing the beneficial bacteria in your water supply and, if unimpeded, within your body.

It's their job to deliver sanitary water to you, but apparently, it's your job to remove the MMM toxins that are put in the water to keep it sanitary as it flows through the sometimes 100-year-old public water system.

A reverse osmosis water filter can also help with removal of many other contaminants that may be in your tap water. These contaminants may include residue from prescription drugs, herbicides, pesticides, viruses, fluoride, heavy metals, plastics in so many forms, and everything else in the environment that settles in or on your water source.

Reverse osmosis is such a great process for clearing microcontaminants from water that it also removes minerals from the water. A sophisticated multivitamin with a trace mineral complex or a separate trace mineral formula helps keep your body's trace mineral levels balanced.

Oral Health

Today I went to the dentist for my regular cleaning. At my appointment four months ago, I presented with significant bleeding of my gums, and they appeared red, puffy, and friable. So rather than my normal six-month period between cleanings, my dentist recommended I return in three-four months for more frequent plaque removal and to keep an eye on my gum health. He said that a buildup of plaque causes inflammation of the gums.

After working for 10-15 minutes, my dental hygienist finally commented that my gums looked so much better than last time and there was no blood or inflammation at all during the cleaning.

She asked if I was doing anything differently. I told her I

developed a new oral product specifically for gum health and within just a few days of taking it with colostrum twice daily after brushing my teeth, my gums and my intestinal inflammation had improved noticeably. I proudly brought the new bottle with me, and she saw that it was titled M-ENT Probiotics. I also told her that a month later I got a water pick cleaner. Her comment was that water picks are very helpful for gum health.

She also did a probing, measuring the depth of the pocket between your gums and your teeth. Today, there were a lot of measurements of 1-3 mm depth, whereas the last probing (done by the same person) showed depth of 3-5 mm throughout my mouth, with one measurement of 6 mm. I was extraordinarily impressed with the apparent improvement in my gum health.

My dentist stopped by during my cleaning and the hygienist relayed the changes to him. He concluded that a water pick is very effective against gum deterioration, apparently even able to work its magic during the month before I bought it, when my only change was taking my new Probiotic lozenge with colostrum.

I thought it was remarkable how indoctrinated and closed minded a dental school graduate may be. After he walked away, I was offered the standard fluoride treatment. I declined as always.

I was offered a little package of a new toothbrush and a sample of the newest name-brand fluoridated toothpaste with saccharin, and the warning to call a poison control center if swallowed. How reassuring!

I left the office thinking how happy I was with validation of the significant improvement of my gum health, how happy I was with the possibility of anecdotal evidence of the plasma (blood) pathway of probiotics through inflamed gum tissue and sublingually to the GI tract, and how disappointed I was with the closed mindedness and dogma that the dentist displayed. He only heard or listened to the part of what I said that he already knew; he couldn't even acknowledge that I was presenting something to think about or that he disagreed with.

Remove and Protect Against Toxic Chemicals

Probiotics may be used for detoxification!

Ultimately our body's elaborate and sophisticated detoxification systems become overloaded, which leads to the emergence of acute and chronic conditions – conditions that conventional medicine frequently diagnose as some kind of disease. Environmental toxicity is not well established as a cause of disease, especially its effect on the MMM. Thus these "diseases" are treated by suppressing symptoms of the body's response to poisoning with patented drugs and pharmaceutical biologics.

Certain beneficial bacteria and yeast – which we co-evolved with and have formed symbiotic alliances with – numbering in the trillions, have been shown in published scientific studies to bind, degrade, and remove specific toxins.

These probiotics can degrade and detoxify the following toxins:

- Perchlorate detox – Perchlorate is a component in jet fuel and fireworks that extensively contaminates the air and our food. It's now found in disturbing amounts in breast milk and urine. Perchlorate is a well-known endocrine disrupter with the ability to block iodine receptors in the thyroid, contributing to hypothyroidism and attendant neurological dysfunction. A recent study found the bacterial strain *Bifidobacterium bifidum* is able to degrade perchlorate, and that breast fed babies appear to have lower levels of perchlorate than formula fed babies. This is due to beneficial bacteria in mother's milk, but not in formula, being able to degrade perchlorate through the perchlorate reductase pathway.[2]

- Pesticide detox – Lactic acid bacterial strains isolated from kimchi, the Korean fermented cabbage dish, have been shown to degrade four different organophosphorus insecticides. These lactic acid strains use these insecticides as a source of carbon and phosphorus.[3,4]

- Bisphenol-A (BPA) detox – Bisphenol A has become a ubiquitous toxicant derived from petrochemicals. BPA has endocrine-disrupting properties. It has been shown to accumulate in the food chain, at the top of which are humans. BPA has been linked to a wide range of health problems. *Bifidobacterium breve* and *Lactobacillus casei* have been demonstrated in animal models to both reduce the intestinal absorption of BPA and enhance its excretion.[5]

- Heavy Metal detox – includes arsenic, cadmium, lead, mercury, and nickel. Heavy metals pose a threat to human health because they can easily enter the body through the skin, respiratory tract, and gastrointestinal tract, all protected by the MMM, and have been associated with adverse health effects, including immune system suppression, hormonal dysregulation, and gut dysbiosis.[6,7] Several strains of *Lactobacillus* have demonstrated the capacity to effectively bind to and sequester heavy metals from water and in

animal cell models.[8] [9-11] *Lactobacillus casei, Lactobacillus plantarum*, and *Lactobacillus rhamnosus* are called out in the studies.[8 9-11]

While Fluoride in public water systems and toothpaste is not a metal, fluoride additives contain heavy metal contaminants that must be diluted to meet drinking water regulations. Heavy metal content varies by batch, and all samples in one study contained arsenic (4.9–56.0 ppm) or arsenic in addition to lead (10.3 ppm).[12] Some samples contained barium (13.3–18.0 ppm) instead. All fluoride samples contained a surprising amount of aluminum. Thus the warning on commercial toothpaste not to swallow it, even though it's pleasantly flavored. This is especially difficult with kids.

Probiotic intervention may reduce plasma heavy metal levels and increase both urinary and fecal excretion. An increased commensal microbial abundance and decreased intestinal permeability has also been shown. Essentially, we see probiotics support the protective mechanisms of the gastrointestinal MMM, thus reducing intestinal permeability to heavy metal toxins. Plus, these probiotics bind to the heavy metals to promote excretion of the toxins. [8 9-11]

- Gluten detox – Wheat and gluten have increasingly been linked as a contributing factor in a wide range of health problems, with up to 300 potential adverse effects identified. *Bifidobacteria* may reduce the immunotoxic properties of gluten peptides by degrading them into non-toxic peptides.[13] Interestingly, the mouth has lately been found to contain bacteria capable of degrading gluten, indicating there may be other gluten-degrading microorganisms within the upper gastrointestinal tract. Something as simple as what your

  mother told you, such as to completely chew your food, may

reduce the potential antigenicity/ immunotoxicity of wheat gluten peptides.[14]

• Aspirin detox – Pharmaceutical companies and some doctors recommend drugs such as aspirin for its preventive role in heart disease, despite the fact that even low-dose aspirin causes intestinal injury and other serious adverse health effects. Though aspirin's adverse health effects have been established in the literature to far outweigh its purported health benefits, millions take it daily without full knowledge of how it's affecting them. The bacteria *Lactobacillus casei* has been shown to reduce damage to the MMM and gastrointestinal tract done by aspirin.[15] Thus you can take *Lactobacillus casei* to reduce side effects of aspirin, even though there are much better means to keep your blood flowing, such as Japanese fermented cheese natto and supplements containing nattokinase.

• Sodium Nitrate detox – Numerous foods are preserved with nitrates, which may form DNA-damaging nitrosamines. Kimchi-derived Lactic acid bacteria have been shown to degrade sodium nitrate.[16]

• Vaccine detox – there is a lot of controversial literature describing the unintended adverse side effects of vaccines. Studies reporting side effects are usually not sponsored by the pharmaceutical companies which market the vaccines. This is especially true for attenuated live vaccines, such as oral polio vaccine, which have lately been linked to thousands of cases of childhood vaccine-induced paralysis in countries such as India. Oral *Saccharomyces boulardii*, a beneficial form of yeast, has been shown in a recent animal study to prevent oral polio vaccine-induced IgA nephropathy, a form of immune-mediated kidney damage.[16] Also, probiotic bacteria have been shown to positively regulate the two poles of immunity (TH1/ TH2), which vaccines frequently upset by inducing hypersensitization via over-activation of the adaptive/humoral (TH2) pole of immunity.[17]

- Chemotherapy detox – No chemical therapy is more fraught with life-changing risks than chemotherapy – used to treat already very sick and weak patients. Some chemotherapy agents, such as the nitrogen mustard class, are so poisonous that they bear chemical munitions designations, and are banned by the Chemical Weapons Convention. There's evidence that the probiotic *Bifidobacterium breve* is able to reduce the adverse effects on immune health induced by chemotherapy agents.[18]

In summary, detox probiotics include:

- *Bifidobacterium bifidum*
- *Bifidobacterium breve*
- *Lactobacillus casei*
- *Lactobacillus plantarum*
- *Lactobacillus rhamnosus*
- *Bifidobacteria*
- Lactic acid bacteria
- *Saccharomyces boulardii*

Other Supplement Recommendations for Environmental Contaminants

Supplements recommended by a founder of the Environmental Health Symposium (EHS) and Garry Gordon, MD:[19]

- A Micro-Contaminant Detox Formula (containing EDTA, N-acetylcholine, chlorella, turmeric, modified citrus pectin, garlic, and broccoli sprouts) to support slow heavy metal chelation and support the liver in clearing many other microcontaminants. Doctors attending EHS have responded that oral chelation is especially appropriate for preventive/prophylactic use as well as maintenance use after intravenous (IV) chelation, or for missed IV chelation appointments.

- In his writings, Garry Gordon MD recommends using a sophisticated multivitamin in conjunction with chelation therapy because the chelation therapy will remove beneficial minerals in addition to environmental contaminants.

Supplements recommended by the late Walter Crinnion, ND, Cofounder of the Environmental Health Symposium:

- Dr. Crinnion once told me, "Howard, your multivitamin has a great combination of what I call "anti-toxicants" and would be a perfect fit for our community." A sophisticated multivitamin is a great adjunct to Micro-Contaminant Detox Formula to support healthy vitamin and mineral levels during detox.[24]

- Dr. Crinnion also said, "I would encourage you to highlight Curcumin and the Colon Cleanse (hardly anyone has good fibers now), in a section of your product display to deal with pollutant overload."[24]

Increase Microbial Diversity in your MMM

The Human Microbiome Project, a global initiative, estimates that the microorganisms that live inside or on humans outnumber body cells by a factor of ten. Only about 1% of this microbiota has been characterized and identified.[20]

Is the goal to overpopulate with one inexpensive strain? No. The goal is to increase the remarkable diversity of beneficial bacteria in the body so that your MMM can use its innate and highly intelligent ability to manage the balance of bacteria in each of the areas in your body. Bacteria work as a community, adapting to the different environments and needs of different body systems and organs.

An analogy is building a house. If you had only plumbers build your house, it might be made out of pipes. If you had only cabinet makers build your house, it would be very compartmentalized. If you had only roofers build your house, at least it wouldn't leak. Sure, they can each do rudimentary work of another trade, but it takes a diversity of trades, starting with an architect, building and soil engineers, foundation experts, framers, plumbers, electricians, tile setters, HVAC experts, and so many more.

Research published in April 2023 in the journal Nature Aging shows that the gut microbiomes of centenarians, people who live the longest, have the most bacteria associated with youth. [23]

Although the study was limited because it was confined to a community in Guangxi, China, the sample size was large: 1,575 people age 20 to 117, 297 people over 100, 301 people aged 90 to 99, 386 people aged 66 to 85, 277 people aged 45 to 65 and 314 people aged 20 to 44 were the groups for this study.

Diversity of gut microbiota was shown to be important for maintaining youthful stability. A portion of the study showed that centenarians with the most diverse species had little change in their gut microbiomes during 18 months of the longitudinal portion. Centenarians also have unique biomarkers; 29 biochemical signatures were found, marking characteristics common in centenarians.

The researchers wrote: "Compared to their old adult counterparts, centenarians displayed youth-associated features in the gut microbiome characterized by an over-representation of a Bacteroides-dominated enterotype, increase in species evenness (diversity), enrichment of potentially beneficial Bacteroidetes and depletion of potential pathobionts."

The differences in gut microbiota across the ages and the link between gut microbiota and health imply that gut microbiome health is associated with longevity for centenarians. It is likely that most centenarians in this study never lost their youthful healthy microbiome. Eating habits, environment, and other personal factors keep the gut microbiota young.[23]

Choose a diversity probiotic formula from an assortment of the most widely available *Lactobacillus*, *Bifidobacteria*, and *Streptococcus* strains, as well as soil-based organisms, *Saccharomyces Boulardii*, and a multitude of trace strains from fermented foods and soil. Fermented foods and soil organisms are the way probiotics were available to mammals long ago. They are still beneficial.

These specific strains identified in our research increase bacterial diversity:

- *Lactobacillus acidophilus*
- *Bifidobacterium lactis*
- *Lactobacillus plantarum*
- *Lactobacillus casei*
- *Lactobacillus rhamnosus*
- *Lactobacillus paracasei*
- *Bifidobacterium breve*
- *Streptococcus thermophilus*
- *Lactobacillus salivarius*
- *Bifidobacterium longum*

Additional diversity is provided by:

- *Saccharomyces boulardii*
- *Bifidobacterium bifidum/Bifidobacterium lactis*
- *Lactobacillus bulgaricus*
- Probiotics from fermented foods and soil

Specific oral bacteria include:

- *Streptococcus salivarius K12*

Colostrum is Superfood for the MMM

Colostrum is the first "milk" produced by the mother of a newborn, whether that mother is human, a cow, or another mammal. It is generally produced by the mother for a period of 48 to 72 hours after giving birth.[21]

Colostrum is the only superfood produced by humans and other mammals. It is the sole source and complete nutrition for a newborn baby containing over 200 bioactive compounds.

These compounds include peptides, defensive antibodies, prebiotics, amino acids, trace minerals, immunoglobulins, tissue growth factors, antioxidants, and other natural immune support that work synergistically to enhance health of the newborn.

There are over 5,000 published studies reporting the benefits of colostrum at all ages.

For children and adults, it provides the magic when taken with a diverse dose of probiotics. Colostrum works synergistically with commensal bacteria (probiotics) to enhance the integrity of the MMM and normal immune function, providing multiple applications – in the GI tract and elsewhere in the body. It helps maintain a robust MMM.

Immunoglobulins

Immunoglobulins like IgG are antibodies that are present in the bloodstream, but also play an important part in the MMM. They can bind to environmental toxins like viruses and bacteria to block them from crossing the MMM and epithelial barriers. They play an integral part in the baby's first-line immune response.[21]

Secretory Immunoglobulin A

Secretory immunoglobulin A (SigA) is the most abundant antibody at epithelial tissue in the respiratory and gastrointestinal tract and plays a pivotal part in immunity. SigA is considered antiviral and antibacterial because it binds and neutralizes viruses and bacteria, precluding them from reaching the tissue. SigA also intercepts allergens and toxins. SigA plays an important role in maintaining homeostasis of gut bacteria (the MMM or microbiome).[21]

Milk Oligosaccharides

Milk oligosaccharides are unique prebiotics only found in colostrum. They pass undigested through the GI tract to reach the large intestine where they serve as a food source for bacteria and feed the whole body MMM. Unlike other prebiotics, milk oligosaccharides have been shown to preferentially feed the bifido-species, supporting balance of good and harmful bacteria in the MMM. Milk oligosaccharides also support beneficial mucous to protect the tissue barrier.[21]

Lactoferrin

Lactoferrin acts as a first line defense against environmental contaminants through several mechanisms. It can bind directly to toxins to destroy them, can block them, may retain other immune cells when trouble is perceived, and is also suitable to induce an anti-inflammatory response. Lactoferrin has been shown to have a strong anti-viral effect against influenza. It also supports zonulin to maintain a tight seal between cells of epithelial tissue.[21]

Human Growth Factors

Human growth factors are proteins that promote cellular rejuvenation and tissue repair. Colostrum is a potent source of growth factors and has been shown to have important efficacy in mending injuries, building muscle, and maintaining skin softness and elasticity. Colostrum is the only natural source of transforming growth factors alpha and beta (TGF-a, TGF-b) and insulin-like growth factors 1 and 2 (IGF- 1, IGF- 2). IGF- 1 from colostrum increases lean muscle and when used during exercise, switches cellular energy from sugar to fat, adding to the body's fat-burning capacity.[21]

World Renowned Expert

Andrew Keech, PhD provides a remarkable discussion of colostrum and peptide Immunotherapy in his 400-page definitive guide to colostrum. He discusses the benefits of colostrum for intestinal permeability, leaky gut syndrome, immune health, diabetes, autoimmune conditions, autism, heart disease, influenza, cancer, AIDS, athletic use, fitness, anti-aging, detoxification, weight loss, tissue repair, injury recovery, and topical applications. All these benefits and conditions support MMM Theory.[21]

Proline-rich polypeptides (PRPs) have been extensively studied for their remarkably varied immune-modulating effect. Researchers have established that the symphony of peptides, all working together, seems to display great synergy. PRP-rich bovine colostrum may have natural immune benefits surpassing those of prescription drugs. PRPs have been shown to help combat numerous kinds of infections and to help autoimmune conditions such as allergies and asthma — in modulating our immune system.

PRPs from bovine colostrum are perceived to induce production of cytokines similar to interferon (IFN) and tumor necrosis factor (TNF) in human leukocytes and in whole blood. The effect is dose related. Experimenters concluded that PRPs may have immunomodulatory value as neurotropic cytokines, one that influences neurological function.[22] In another study, PRPs stimulated interferon (IFN) and tumor necrosis factor (TNF) peritoneal cells from mice, by over 30-times.

A robust immune response needs to be aggressive and indeed inflammatory in the acute phase of attack, then quickly relent, to heal any leftover inflammation. That's what PRPs help our system to do. A 2008 study of allergic responses showed that PRPs from mother's milk colostrum significantly reduced production of IgE/ IgG1, airway eosinophilia, mucin, and down-regulated hypersensitivity — all initiated by allergenic compounds from ragweed pollen grains and house dust. The experimenters concluded that PRPs are effective in precluding allergic responses to many allergens.

Colostrum uniquely contains lactoferrin, immunoglobulins, and PRPs. Bovine colostrum (from cows) is 40 times richer in immune factors than human colostrum. Bovine colostrum is biologically suitable for humans. Look for colostrum that contains no recombinant bovine growth hormones (rBGH), is concentrated to contain 30% immunoglobulins, and collected within the first 12 hours after birthing to ensure the highest concentration of these healthy nutrients.

Supporting the Respiratory MMM

The respiratory system is highly complex. It provides the body with oxygen (O_2) and simultaneously expels carbon dioxide (CO_2). It protects against entry of airborne microcontaminants and helps expel microcontaminants.

MMM Theory posits that the intelligent differentiation between nutrients such as oxygen and waste such as carbon dioxide and microcontaminants is managed by the respiratory microbiome.

We believe you can support your respiratory microbiome with inhalation of a mixture of beneficial bacteria (probiotics) and colostrum. A couple of capsules of a diverse mix of probiotics and a pinch of colostrum may be mixed in clean (sterilized or reverse osmosis) water. Then aerosolized and inhaled into the sinuses. This home-made formula may be kept in the refrigerator for a week or so, once the freeze-dried probiotics are mixed with water.

Supporting the Skin MMM

The dermal or skin MMM is highly complex and located on the surface of your skin as well as within the dermal layer. It is made up of a variety of beneficial bacteria as we describe in Chapter 8 - skin microbiome.

Conditions that can benefit from a healthier MMM include acne, psoriasis, itching, hair health, "autoimmune diseases" of the skin, underarm odor, and others.

The simplest way to support your dermal MMM is to apply a solution to your skin consisting of distilled or reverse osmosis water, a couple of capsules of a diverse probiotic blend, a pinch of colostrum roughly equal to the volume of probiotics in the capsules you use, and twice the amount of whey protein powder. Mix these in a small bottle with a cap that you keep refrigerated after mixing the solution. Dab a few drops on the area you want to protect after washing.

Dr. Meletis described his pajama therapy in Chapter 8. Given two patients, one healthy and one with a skin issue, the healthy subject sleeps in pajamas for a few nights, then without washing the pajamas, the patient with a skin problem wears the pajamas for a few nights. Effectively, this acts as a skin microbiome transplant from the healthy patient to the dysbiotic patient. The pajamas should then be thoroughly washed, and the procedure repeated.

Treatment with Antibiotics

Antibiotics are designed and used to kill bacteria. Some antibiotics are more targeted than others. All have a warning that side effects include stomach and intestinal issues can present up to months after taking the antibiotics.

In order to maintain some of the beneficial bacteria in your MMM concurrently with antibiotic use and restore your MMM after antibiotic use, we recommend repopulating your MMM in your gut and elsewhere with probiotics taken for a few months after antibiotic use.

For this purpose, a diversity of strains, such as 10 or more strains, is recommended. Sporing strains such as S. *Boulardii* are also recommended.

Although medical dogma says that you need to take the antibiotics for their full course, we suggest that is not always necessary. We consider the goal of antibiotic therapy to be to destroy most of the harmful bacteria and insist that it must include restoring a balance of beneficial and harmful bacteria that will always coexist in your body. It may not be necessary to wipe out every last harmful bacterium or the entire microbiome in order to return the body and the MMM to homeostasis, a balanced state.

Conclusion

You have a great deal of choices – some are easy, others are extremely difficult. They include the food you eat, the environment in which you live, the work which you do, the water you drink and bathe in, the model of your cell phone and how you use it and other electronic devices, the way you treat a health issue, and the support you provide your body and your synergistic microbial mucosal milieu (MMM).

Choose wisely to promote a long and healthy life!

For scientists, researchers, and physicians, there is so much yet to understand about the human condition and our connection with bacteria and our environment. Keep an open mind and seek the little clues which guide you to question medical and pharmaceutical dogma.

We hope this book has led you to a greater appreciation for the human and animal MMM and that it may be a key to human health and healthy longevity.

Chapter One References

1. www.niehs.nih.gov/health/topics/conditions/ inflammation/index.cfm (Accessed Nov. 2022)

2. Aagaard K, Ma J, Antony KM, Ganu R, Petrosino J, Versalovic J. (2014) The placenta harbors a unique microbiome. *Sci Transl Med.* May 21;6(237),

3. Song, S. J., Lauber, C., Costello, E. K., Lozupone, C. A., Humphrey, G., Berg-Lyons, D., Caporaso, J. G., Knights, D., Clemente, J. C., Nakielny, S., Gordon, J. I., Fierer, N., & Knight, R. (2012). Cohabiting family members share microbiota with one another and with their dogs. *eLife*, 2.

4. Mireya UA, Martí PO, Xavier KV, Cristina LO, Miguel MM, Magda CM. (2007) Nosocomial infections in paediatric and neonatal intensive care units. J *Infect. Mar*;54(3):212-20.

5. Combellick JL, Shin H, Shin D, Cai Y, Hagan H, Lacher C, Lin DL, McCauley K, Lynch SV, Dominguez-Bello MG. (2018) Differences in the fecal microbiota of neonates born at home or in the hospital. *Sci Rep.* Oct 23;8(1):15660.

6. Hölscher B, Frye C, Wichmann HE, Heinrich J. Exposure to pets and allergies in children. *Pediatr Allergy Immunol.* 2002 Oct;13(5):334-41.

7. Gilbert, J.A. Our unique microbial identity. (2015) *Genome Biol* 16, 97.

8. Soderborg TK, Clark SE, Mulligan CE, Janssen RC, Babcock L, Ir D, Young B, Krebs N, Lemas DJ, Johnson LK, Weir T, Lenz LL, Frank DN, Hernandez TL, Kuhn KA, D'Alessandro A, Barbour LA, El Kasmi KC, Friedman JE. (2018) The gut microbiota in infants of obese mothers increases inflammation and

susceptibility to NAFLD. *Nat Commun.* Oct 26;9(1):4462.

9. Li S, Song J, Ke P, Kong L, Lei B, Zhou J, Huang Y, Li H, Li G, Chen J, Li X, Xiang Z, Ning Y, Wu F, Wu K. (2021) The gut microbiome is associated with brain structure and function in schizophrenia. *Sci Rep.* May 7;11(1):9743.

10. Kolodziejczyk AA, Zheng D, Elinav E. (2019) Diet-microbiota interactions and personalized nutrition. *Nat Rev Microbiol.* Dec;17(12):742-753.

11. Obrenovich MEM. (2018) Leaky Gut, Leaky Brain? Microorganisms. Oct 18;6(4):107.

12. Wilson, A. S., Koller, K. R., Ramaboli, M. C., Nesengani, L. T., Ocvirk, S., Chen, C., Flanagan, C. A., Sapp, F. R., Merritt, Z. T., Bhatti, F., & Thomas, T. K. (2020). Diet and the Human Gut Microbiome: An International Review. *Digestive diseases and sciences*, 65(3), 723.

13. Singh, R. K., Chang, W., Yan, D., Lee, K. M., Ucmak, D., Wong, K., Abrouk, M., Farahnik, B., Nakamura, M., Zhu, T. H., Bhutani, T., & Liao, W. (2016). Influence of diet on the gut microbiome and implications for human health. *Journal of Translational Medicine*, 15.

14. David LA, Maurice CF, Carmody RN, Gootenberg DB, Button JE, Wolfe BE, Ling AV, Devlin AS, Varma Y, Fischbach MA, Biddinger SB, Dutton RJ, Turnbaugh PJ. (2014) Diet rapidly and reproducibly alters the human gut microbiome. *Nature.* Jan 23;505(7484):559-63.

15. Ames BN (2006) Low micronutrient intake may accelerate the degenerative diseases of aging through allocation of scarce micronutrients by triage. *Proc. Natl. Acad. Sciences*

USA, 103:17589-94.

16. Ames BN. Prevention of mutation, cancer, and other age-associated diseases by optimizing micronutrient intake. *J of Nucleic Acids*; rev. July 28, 2010; in press.

Chapter Two References

1. Pizzorno J. *The Toxin Solution: How Hidden Poisons in the Air, Water, Food, and Products We Use Are Destroying Our Health--AND WHAT WE CAN DO TO FIX IT* HarperOne; 2017.

2. Krüger M, Shehata AA, Schrödl W, Rodloff A. Glyphosate suppresses the antagonistic effect of Enterococcus spp. on Clostridium botulinum. *Anaerobe.* 2013;20:74-78.

3. Shehata AA, Schrödl W, Aldin AA, Hafez HM, Krüger M. The effect of glyphosate on potential pathogens and beneficial members of poultry microbiota in vitro. *Curr Microbiol.* 2013;66(4):350-358.

4. Samsel A. Glyphosate's Suppression of Cytochrome P450 Enzymes and Amino Acid Biosynthesis by the Gut Microbiome: Pathways to Modern Diseases *Entropy.* 2013;15(4).

5. Krivić H, Himbert S, Sun R, Feigis M, Rheinstädter MC. Erythro-PmBs: A Selective Polymyxin B Delivery System Using Antibody-Conjugated Hybrid Erythrocyte Liposomes. *ACS Infect Dis.* 2022;8(10):2059-2072.

6. Chloramines in Drinking Water. EPA. https://www.epa.gov/dwreginfo/chloramines-drinking-water. Published 2022. Updated April 18, 2022. Accessed November 22, 2022.

7. Chloramines and Pool Operation. CDC. https://www.cdc.gov/healthywater/swimming/aquatics-professionals/chloramines.html. Published 2022. Accessed November 23, 2022.

8. News C. EWG's "Hall of Shame" of toxic household cleaners. CBS News. https://www.cbsnews.com/pictures/ewgs-hall-

of-shame-of-toxic-household-cleaners/. Published 2012. Accessed November 23, 2022.

9. Ji Y, Azuine RE, Zhang Y, et al. Association of Cord Plasma Biomarkers of In Utero Acetaminophen Exposure With Risk of Attention-Deficit/Hyperactivity Disorder and Autism Spectrum Disorder in Childhood. JAMA *Psychiatry*. 2020;77(2):180-189.

10. Weil J, Colin-Jones D, Langman M, et al. Prophylactic aspirin and risk of peptic ulcer bleeding. *Bmj*. 1995;310(6983):827-830.

11. Kelly JP, Kaufman DW, Jurgelon JM, Sheehan J, Koff RS, Shapiro S. Risk of aspirin-associated major upper-gastrointestinal bleeding with enteric-coated or buffered product. *Lancet*. 1996;348(9039):1413-1416.

12. Mullenix PJ. A new perspective on metals and other contaminants in fluoridation chemicals. *Int J Occup Environ Health*. 2014;20(2):157-166.

13. Monachese M, Burton JP, Reid G. Bioremediation and tolerance of humans to heavy metals through microbial processes: a potential role for probiotics? *Appl Environ Microbiol*. 2012;78(18):6397-6404.

14. Daisley BA, Monachese M, Trinder M, et al. Immobilization of cadmium and lead by Lactobacillus rhamnosus GR-1 mitigates apical-to-basolateral heavy metal translocation in a Caco-2 model of the intestinal epithelium. *Gut Microbes*. 2019;10(3):321-333.

15. Chen Z, Tang Z, Kong J, et al. Lactobacillus casei SYF-08 Protects Against Pb-Induced Injury in Young Mice by

Regulating Bile Acid Metabolism and Increasing Pb Excretion. *Front Nutr.* 2022;9:914323.

16. Zhai Q, Liu Y, Wang C, et al. Lactobacillus plantarum CCFM8661 modulates bile acid enterohepatic circulation and increases lead excretion in mice. *Food Funct.* 2019;10(3):1455-1464.

17. Zhai Q, Tian F, Zhao J, Zhang H, Narbad A, Chen W. Oral Administration of Probiotics Inhibits Absorption of the Heavy Metal Cadmium by Protecting the Intestinal Barrier. *Appl Environ Microbiol.* 2016;82(14):4429-4440.

18. Lentini P, Zanoli L, Granata A, Signorelli SS, Castellino P, Dell'Aquila R. Kidney and heavy metals - The role of environmental exposure (Review). *Mol Med Rep.* 2017;15(5):3413-3419.

19. García-Niño WR, Pedraza-Chaverrí J. Protective effect of curcumin against heavy metals-induced liver damage. *Food Chem Toxicol.* 2014;69:182-201.

20. Bakulski KM, Seo YA, Hickman RC, et al. Heavy Metals Exposure and Alzheimer's Disease and Related Dementias. *J Alzheimers Dis.* 2020;76(4):1215-1242.

21. Zhai Q, Liu Y, Wang C, et al. Increased Cadmium Excretion Due to Oral Administration of Lactobacillus plantarum Strains by Regulating Enterohepatic Circulation in Mice. *J Agric Food Chem.* 2019;67(14):3956-3965.

22. Shelor CP, Kirk AB, Dasgupta PK, Kroll M, Campbell CA, Choudhary PK. Breastfed infants metabolize perchlorate. *Environ Sci Technol.* 2012;46(9):5151-5159.

23. Cho KM, Math RK, Islam SM, et al. Biodegradation of chlorpyrifos by lactic acid bacteria during kimchi

fermentation. *J Agric Food Chem.* 2009;57(5):1882-1889.

24. Islam SM, Math RK, Cho KM, et al. Organophosphorus hydrolase (OpdB) of Lactobacillus brevis WCP902 from kimchi is able to degrade organophosphorus pesticides. *J Agric Food Chem.* 2010;58(9):5380-5386.

25. Oishi K, Sato T, Yokoi W, Yoshida Y, Ito M, Sawada H. Effect of probiotics, Bifidobacterium breve and Lactobacillus casei, on bisphenol A exposure in rats. *Biosci Biotechnol Biochem.* 2008;72(6):1409-1415.

26. Laparra JM, Sanz Y. Bifidobacteria inhibit the inflammatory response induced by gliadins in intestinal epithelial cells via modifications of toxic peptide generation during digestion. *J Cell Biochem.* 2010;109(4):801-807.

27. Helmerhorst EJ, Zamakhchari M, Schuppan D, Oppenheim FG. Discovery of a novel and rich source of gluten-degrading microbial enzymes in the oral cavity. *PLoS One.* 2010;5(10):e13264.

28. Endo H, Higurashi T, Hosono K, et al. Efficacy of Lactobacillus casei treatment on small bowel injury in chronic low-dose aspirin users: a pilot randomized controlled study. *J Gastroenterol.* 2011;46(7):894-905.

29. Ralph E. Holsworth J, D.O. Healthy Blood Circulation with Nattokinase. https://www.rejuvenation-science.com/nattokinase. Accessed November 23, 2022.

30. Oh CK, Oh MC, Kim SH. The depletion of sodium nitrite by lactic acid bacteria isolated from kimchi. *J Med Food.* 2004;7(1):38-44.

31. Soylu A, Berktaş S, Sarioğlu S, et al. Saccharomyces boulardii

prevents oral-poliovirus vaccine-induced IgA nephropathy in mice. *Pediatr Nephrol.* 2008;23(8):1287-1291.

32. Tan M, Zhu JC, Du J, Zhang LM, Yin HH. Effects of probiotics on serum levels of Th1/Th2 cytokine and clinical outcomes in severe traumatic brain-injured patients: a prospective randomized pilot study. *Crit Care.* 2011;15(6):R290.

33. Wada M, Nagata S, Saito M, et al. Effects of the enteral administration of Bifidobacterium breve on patients undergoing chemotherapy for pediatric malignancies. *Support Care Cancer.* 2010;18(6):751-759.

34. O.T. W. The Effects of anthropogenic EMF on biological organisms. https://committees.parliament.uk/writtenevidence/1794/html/. Accessed November 23, 2022.

35. Keulers L, Dehghani A, Knippels L, et al. Probiotics, prebiotics, and synbiotics to prevent or combat air pollution consequences: The gut-lung axis. *Environ Pollut.* 2022;302:119066.

Chapter Three References

1. Thomas RM, Jobin C. Microbiota in pancreatic health and disease: the next frontier in microbiome research. *Nat Rev Gastroenterol Hepatol.* 2020;17(1):53-64.

2. Wei MY, Shi S, Liang C, et al. The microbiota and microbiome in pancreatic cancer: more influential than expected. *Mol Cancer.* 2019;18(1):97.

3. Clifford A, Hoffman GS. Evidence for a vascular microbiome and its role in vessel health and disease. *Curr Opin Rheumatol.* 2015;27(4):397-405.

4. Tariq S, Clifford AH. An update on the microbiome in vasculitis. *Curr Opin Rheumatol.* 2021;33(1):15-23.

5. Reitsma S, Slaaf DW, Vink H, van Zandvoort MA, oude Egbrink MG. The endothelial glycocalyx: composition, functions, and visualization. *Pflugers Arch.* 2007;454(3):345-359.

6. Yu Y, Liu B, Liu X, et al. Mesenteric lymph system constitutes the second route in gut-liver axis and transports metabolism-modulating gut microbial metabolites. *J Genet Genomics.* 2022;49(7):612-623.

7. Leinwand JC, Paul B, Chen R, et al. Intrahepatic microbes govern liver immunity by programming NKT cells. *J Clin Invest.* 2022;132(8).

8. Suppli MP, Bagger JI, Lelouvier B, et al. Hepatic microbiome in healthy lean and obese humans. JHEP Rep. 2021;3(4):100299.

9. Aagaard K, Ma J, Antony KM, Ganu R, Petrosino J, Versalovic J. The placenta harbors a unique microbiome. *Sci Transl Med.* 2014;6(237):237ra265.

10. Younge N, McCann JR, Ballard J, et al. Fetal exposure to the maternal microbiota in humans and mice. *JCI Insight*. 2019;4(19).

11. Pohl HG, Groah SL, Pérez-Losada M, et al. The Urine Microbiome of Healthy Men and Women Differs by Urine Collection Method. *Int Neurourol J.* 2020;24(1):41-51.

12. Gottschick C, Deng ZL, Vital M, et al. The urinary microbiota of men and women and its changes in women during bacterial vaginosis and antibiotic treatment. *Microbiome*. 2017;5(1):99.

13. Dai D, Yang Y, Yang Y, et al. Alterations of thyroid microbiota across different thyroid microhabitats in patients with thyroid carcinoma. *J Transl Med*. 2021;19(1):488.

14. Link C. Is there a brain microbiome? *Neuroscience Insights*. 2021.

15. Berthelot JM, Sellam J, Maugars Y, Berenbaum F. Cartilage-gut-microbiome axis: a new paradigm for novel therapeutic opportunities in osteoarthritis. *RMD Open*. 2019;5(2):e001037.

16. Rohde H. Question 18: Is there a distinct microbiome in the joints? https://www.ors.org/wp-content/uploads/2019/01/Question-18.pdf. Accessed.

17. Verstraelen H, Vieira-Baptista P, De Seta F, Ventolini G, Lonnee-Hoffmann R, Lev-Sagie A. The Vaginal Microbiome: I. Research Development, Lexicon, Defining "Normal" and the Dynamics Throughout Women's Lives. *J Low Genit Tract Dis*. 2022;26(1):73-78.

18. France M, Alizadeh M, Brown S, Ma B, Ravel J. Towards a deeper understanding of the vaginal microbiota. *Nat Microbiol*. 2022;7(3):367-378.

19. Franco-Obregón A, Gilbert JA. The Microbiome-Mitochondrion Connection: Common Ancestries, Common Mechanisms, Common Goals. *mSystems*. 2017;2(3).

20. Castillo DJ, Rifkin RF, Cowan DA, Potgieter M. The Healthy Human Blood Microbiome: Fact or Fiction? *Front Cell Infect Microbiol*. 2019;9:148.

21. Liu Y, Xiao F, Zhang R, Zhang X. Alterations of Plasma Microbiome: A Potentially New Perspective to the Dysbiosis in Systemic Lupus Erythematosus? *J Rheumatol*. 2022;49(6):549-551.

Chapter Four References

1. Sciences NIoEH. Inflammation. National Institute of Environmental Health Sciences. https://www.niehs.nih.gov/health/topics/conditions/inflammation/index.cfm#footnote1. Accessed November 23, 2022.

2. Sciences NIoEH. Inflammation NIH. https://www.niehs.nih.gov/health/topics/conditions/inflammation/index.cfm. Updated April 28, 2021. Accessed November 25, 2022.

3. Furman D, Campisi J, Verdin E, et al. Chronic inflammation in the etiology of disease across the life span. Nat Med. 2019;25(12):1822-1832.

4. Toxicology in the 21st Century (Tox21). National Toxicology Program. https://ntp.niehs.nih.gov/whatwestudy/tox21/index.html. Published 2020. Accessed November 25, 2022.

Chapter Five References

1. Loer SA, Scheeren TW, Tarnow J. (1997) How much oxygen does the human lung consume? Anesthesiology. Mar;86(3):532-7.

2. www.epa.gov/pm-pollution/particulate-matter-pm-basics#effects (Accessed Nov. 11, 2022)

3. Brändli O. (1996) Sind inhalierte Staubpartikel schädlich für unsere Lungen? [Are inhaled dust particles harmful for our lungs?]. Schweiz Med Wochenschr. Dec 14;126(50):2165-74.

4. Whiteside SA, McGinniss JE, Collman RG. (2021) The lung microbiome: progress and promise. J Clin Invest. Aug 2;131(15):e150473.

5. Dickson RP, Erb-Downward JR, Freeman CM, McCloskey L, Falkowski NR, Huffnagle GB, Curtis JL. (2017) Bacterial Topography of the Healthy Human Lower Respiratory Tract. mBio. Feb 14;8(1):e02287-16.

6. Charlson ES, Bittinger K, Haas AR, Fitzgerald AS, Frank I, Yadav A, Bushman FD, Collman RG. (2011) Topographical continuity of bacterial populations in the healthy human respiratory tract. Am J Respir Crit Care Med. Oct 15;184(8):957-63.

7. Gleeson K, Maxwell SL, Eggli DF. (1997) Quantitative Aspiration During Sleep in Normal Subjects. Chest Journal. 111(5):1255-72.

8. Invernizzi R, Barnett J, Rawal B, Nair A, Ghai P, Kingston S, Chua F, Wu Z, Wells AU, Renzoni ER, Nicholson AG, Rice A, Lloyd CM, Byrne AJ, Maher TM, Devaraj A, Molyneaux PL. (2020) Bacterial burden in the lower airways predicts disease progression in idiopathic pulmonary fibrosis and is independent of radiological disease extent. Eur Respir J. Apr

3;55(4):1901519.

9. Jenerowicz D, et al. (2012) Environmental factors and allergic diseases. *Ann Agric Environ Med.* 19(3):475-81.

10. Xaubet A, et al. (2013) Guidelines for the diagnosis and treatment of idiopathic pulmonary fibrosis. Sociedad Española de Neumología y Cirugía Torácica (SEPAR) Research Group on Diffuse Pulmonary Diseases. *Arch Bronconeumol.* Aug;49(8):343-53.

11. Kandhare AD, et al. (2016) Efficacy of antioxidant in idiopathic pulmonary fibrosis: A systematic review and meta-analysis. *EXCLI J.*Nov 7;15:636-51.

12. Meltzer EB, Noble PW. (2008) Idiopathic pulmonary fibrosis. *Orphanet J Rare Dis.* Mar 26;3:8.

13. Luppi F, et al. (2012) The big clinical trials in idiopathic pulmonary fibrosis. *Curr Opin Pulm Med.* Sep;18(5):428-32.

14. Burke DG, et al. (2017)The altered gut microbiota in adults with cystic fibrosis. *BMC Microbiol.* Mar 9;17(1):58.

15. Cystic Fibrosis Foundation. https://www.cff.org/What-is-CF/About-Cystic-Fibrosis/ Accessed May 4, 2018.

16. Greger R. (2000) Role of CFTR in the colon. *Annu Rev Physiol.* 62:467-91.

17. Manniello MD, et al. (2017) Clarithromycin and N-acetylcysteine co-spray-dried powders for pulmonary drug delivery: A focus on drug solubility. *Int J Pharm.* Nov 30;533(2):463-69.

18. Dhooghe B, et al. (2014) Lung inflammation in cystic fibrosis: pathogenesis and novel therapies. *Clin Biochem.* May;47(7-8):539-46.

19. Sagel SD, Chmiel JF, Konstan MW. (2007) Sputum biomarkers of inflammation in cystic fibrosis lung disease. *Proc Am Thorac Soc.* Aug 1;4(4):406-17.

20. Karp CL, et al. (2004) Defective lipoxin-mediated anti-inflammatory activity in the cystic fibrosis airway. *Nat Immunol.* Apr;5(4):388-92.

21. Freedman SD, et al. (2004) Association of cystic fibrosis with abnormalities in fatty acid metabolism. *N Engl J Med.* Feb 5;350(6):560-9.

22. O'Connor MG, et al. (2016) Elevated prostaglandin E metabolites and abnormal plasma fatty acids at baseline in pediatric cystic fibrosis patients: a pilot study. *Prostaglandins Leukot Essent Fatty Acids.* Oct;113:46-9.

23. Centers for Disease Control andPrevention. https://www.cdc.gov/nchs/fastats/asthma.htm Accessed May 4, 2018.

24. Miller AL. (2001) The etiologies, pathophysiology, and alternative/complementary treatment of asthma. *Altern Med Rev.* Feb;6(1):20-47.

25. Centers for Disease Control and Prevention. https://www.cdc.gov/copd/index.html Accessed May 4, 2018.

26. Valdivieso ÁG, et al. (2018) N-acetyl cysteine reverts the proinflammatory state induced by cigarette smoke extract in lung Calu-3 cells. *Redox Biol.* Jun;16:294-302.

27. Mehta AJ, et al. (2012) Occupational exposure to dusts, gases, and fumes and incidence of chronic obstructive pulmonary disease in the Swiss cohort study on air pollution and lung and heart diseases in adults. *Am J Respir Crit Care Med.* June;185(12):1292-1300.

28. Esquinas C, et al. (2017) Gene and miRNA expression profiles in PBMCs from patients with severe and mild emphysema and PiZZ alpha1-antitrypsin deficiency. *Int J Chron Obstruct Pulmon Dis.* Nov 29;12:3381-90.

29. Millares, L., Pascual, S., Montón, C. et al. (2019)Relationship between the respiratory microbiome and the severity of airflow limitation, history of exacerbations and circulating eosinophils in COPD patients. *BMC Pulm Med* (19) 112.)

30. Mayhew D, Devos N, Lambert C on behalf of the AERIS Study Group et al. (2018) Longitudinal profiling of the lung microbiome in the AERIS study demonstrates repeatability of bacterial and eosinophilic COPD exacerbations *Thorax* 73:422-430.

31. Opron, K., Begley, L.A., Erb-Downward, J.R. et al. (2021) Lung microbiota associations with clinical features of COPD in the SPIROMICS cohort. *npj Biofilms Microbiomes* 7:14.

32. Pragman, A.A., Knutson, K.A., Gould, T.J. et al. (2019) Chronic obstructive pulmonary disease upper airway microbiota alpha diversity is associated with exacerbation phenotype: a case-control observational study. *Respir Res* 20, 114.

33. Moore BB, Moore TA. (2015) Viruses in Idiopathic Pulmonary Fibrosis. Etiology and Exacerbation. *Ann Am Thorac Soc.* Nov; 12(Suppl 2): S186-92.

34. Ueda T, et al. (1992) Idiopathic pulmonary fibrosis and high prevalence of serum antibodies to hepatitis C virus. *Am Rev Respir Dis.* Jul;146(1):266-8.

35. Arase Y, et al. (2008) Hepatitis C virus enhances incidence of idiopathic pulmonary fibrosis. *World J Gastroenterol.* Oct 14;14(38):5880-6.

36. Meliconi R, et al. Incidence of hepatitis C virus infection in Italian patients with idiopathic pulmonary fibrosis. *Thorax.* 1996 Mar; 51(3): 315-17.

37. Lasithiotaki I, et al. (2011) Detection of herpes simplex virus type-1 in patients with fibrotic lung diseases. PLoS One. 6(12):e27800.

38. Pulkkinen V, et al. (2012) A novel screening method detects herpes viral DNA in the idiopathic pulmonary fibrosis lung. *Ann Med.* Mar;44(2):178-86.

39. Tang YW, et al. (2003) Herpesvirus DNA is consistently detected in lungs of patients with idiopathic pulmonary fibrosis. *J Clin Microbiol.* Jun;41(6):2633-40.

40. Lawson WE, et al. (2008) Endoplasmic reticulum stress in alveolar epithelial cells is prominent in IPF: association with altered surfactant protein processing and herpes virus infection. *Am J Physiol Lung Cell Mol Physiol.* Jun;294(6):L1119-26.

41. Calabrese F, et al. (2013) Herpes virus infection is associated with vascular remodeling and pulmonary hypertension in idiopathic pulmonary fibrosis. *PLoS One.* 8(2):e55715.

42. Bando M, et al. (2001) Infection of TT virus in patients with idiopathic pulmonary fibrosis. *Respir Med*. Dec;95(12):935-42.

43. Wootton SC, et al. (2011) Viral infection in acute exacerbation of idiopathic pulmonary fibrosis. *Am J Respir Crit Care Med*. Jun 15;183(12):1698-702.

44. Freer G, et al. (2018) The Virome and Its Major Component, Anellovirus, a Convoluted System Molding Human Immune Defenses and Possibly Affecting the Development of Asthma and Respiratory Diseases in Childhood. *Front Microbiol*. Apr 10;9:686.

45. Strannegård IL, Strannegård O. (1981) Epstein-Barr virus antibodies in children with atopic disease. *Int Arch Allergy Appl Immunol*. 64(3):314-9.

46. Marin J, et al. (2000) Persistence of viruses in upper respiratory tract of children with asthma. *J Infect*. Jul;41(1):69-72.

47. Zheng XY, et al. (2018) Regional, age and respiratory-secretion-specific prevalence of respiratory viruses associated with asthma exacerbation: a literature review. *Arch Virol*. Apr;163(4):845-53,

48. Hahn DL. (1999) Chlamydia pneumoniae, asthma, and COPD: what is the evidence? *Ann Allergy Asthma Immunol*. Oct;83(4):271-88, 291; quiz 291-2.

49. Black PN, et al. (2000) Serological evidence of infection with Chlamydia pneumoniae is related to the severity of asthma. *Eur Respir J*. Feb;15(2):254-9.

50. Fidler L, et al. (2018) Treatment of Gastroesophageal Reflux in Patients With Idiopathic Pulmonary Fibrosis: A Systematic Review and Meta-Analysis. *Chest.* Mar 17.

51. Sontag SJ. (2000) Why do the published data fail to clarify the relationship between gastroesophageal reflux and asthma? *Am J Med.* Mar 6;108 Suppl 4a:159S-69S.

52. Chakrabarti S, et al. (1995) Airway response to acid instillation in esophagus in bronchial asthma. *Indian J Gastroenterol.* Apr;14(2):44-7.

53. Li L, Somerset S. (2014)The clinical significance of the gut microbiota in cystic fibrosis and the potential for dietary therapies. *Clin Nutr.* Aug;33(4):571-80.

54. Burke DG, et al. (2017) The altered gut microbiota in adults with cystic fibrosis. *BMC Microbiol.* Mar 9;17(1):58.

55. Loewen K, et al. (2018) Prenatal antibiotic exposure and childhood asthma: a population-based study. *Eur Respir J.* Apr 20.

56. Okba AM, et al. (2018) Fecal microbiota profile in atopic asthmatic adult patients. *Eur Ann Allergy Clin Immunol.* Jan 15. [Epub ahead of print.]

57. Casaro MC, et al. (2018) Prophylactic Bifidobacterium adolescentis ATTCC 15703 supplementation reduces partially allergic airway disease in Balb/c but not in C57BL/6 mice. *Benef Microbes.* Apr 25;9(3):465-76.

58. Miraglia Del Giudice M, et al. (2012) Airways allergic inflammation and L. reuterii treatment in asthmatic children. *J Biol Regul Homeost Agents.* Jan-Mar;26(1 Suppl):S35-40.

59. Williams NC, et al. (2016) A prebiotic galactooligosaccharide mixture reduces severity of hyperpnoea-induced bronchoconstriction and markers of airway inflammation. *Br J Nutr.* Sep;116(5):798-804.

60. Whyand T, et al. (2018) Pollution and respiratory disease: can diet or supplements help? A review. *Respir Res.* May 2;19(1):79.

61. Conti S, et al. (2018) The association between air pollution and the incidence of idiopathic pulmonary fibrosis in Northern Italy. *Eur Respir J.* Jan 25;51(1).

62. Seymour BW, et al. (1997) Second-hand smoke is an adjuvant for T helper-2 responses in a murine model of allergy. *J Immunol.* Dec 15;159(12):6169-75.

63. Taskar VS, Coultas DB. (2006) Is idiopathic pulmonary fibrosis an environmental disease? *Proc Am Thorac Soc.* Jun;3(4):293-8.

64. Whiteside SA, McGinniss JE, Collman RG. (2021) The Lung Microbiome: Progress and Promise. J Clin Invest. 131(15):e150473.

65. Bahri S, et al. (2017) Prophylactic and curative effect of rosemary leaves extract in a bleomycin model of pulmonary fibrosis. *Pharm Biol.* Dec;55(1):462-71.

66. Yang LT, et al. (2013) [Effects of diterpene phenol extract of Rosmarinus officinalis on TGFbeta1 and mRNA expressions of its signaling pathway molecules in the lung tissue of pulmonary fibrosis rats]. *Zhongguo Zhong xi yi jie he xue hui.* June;33(6):819-24.

67. Bahri S, et al. (2017) Rosmarinic acid potentiates carnosic acid induced apoptosis in lung fibroblasts. *PLoS One*. Sep 6;12(9):e0184368.

68. Kim HR, et al. (2006) Green tea extract inhibits paraquat-induced pulmonary fibrosis by suppression of oxidative stress and endothelin-1 expression. *Lung*. Sep-Oct;184(5):287-95.

69. Hamdy   MA, El-Maraghy   SA, Kortam   MA.   (2012) extract against experimentally induced pulmonaryfibrosis: a comparison with N-acetyl cysteine. *J Biochem Mol Toxicol*. Nov;26(11):461-8.

70. Daba MH, et al. (2002) Effects of L-carnitine and ginkgo biloba extract (EG b 761) in experimental bleomycin-induced lung fibrosis. *Pharmacol Res*. Jun;45(6):461-7.

71. Zhang K, et al. (2016) Preventive Effects of Rhodiola rosea L. on Bleomycin-Induced Pulmonary Fibrosis in Rats. *Int J Mol Sci*. Jun 3;17(6).

72. Wang X, et al. (2018) Buyang Huanwu Decoction Ameliorates Bleomycin-Induced   Pulmonary   Fibrosis   in   Rats   via Downregulation of Related Protein and Gene Expression. *Evid Based Complement Alternat Med*. Feb 28;2018:9185485.

73. Sun T, Liu J, Zhao de W. (2016) Efficacy of N-Acetylcysteine in Idiopathic Pulmonary Fibrosis: A Systematic Review and Meta-Analysis. *Medicine (Baltimore)*. May;95(19):e3629.

74. Homma S, Azuma A, Taniguchi H, et al. (2012) Efficacy of inhaled N-acetylcysteine monotherapy in patients with early stage idiopathic pulmonary fibrosis. *Respirology*. Apr;17(3):467-77.

75. Mimoun M, et al. (2009) Increased tissue arachidonic acid and reduced linoleic acid in a mouse model of cystic fibrosis are reversed by supplemental glycerophospholipids enriched in docosahexaenoic acid. J Nutr. Dec;139(12):2358-64.

76. Hanssens L, et al. (2016) The clinical benefits of long-term supplementation with omega-3 fatty acids in cystic fibrosis patients – A pilot study. Prostaglandins Leukot Essent Fatty Acids. May;108:45-50.

77. Rivas-Crespo MF, et al. (2013) High serum retinol and lung function in young patients with cystic fibrosis. J Pediatr Gastroenterol Nutr. Jun;56(6):657-62.

78. Kelly FJ, et al. (1999) Altered lung antioxidant status in patients with mild asthma. Lancet. Aug 7;354(9177):482-3.

79. Romieu I, et al. (2002) Antioxidant supplementation and lung functions among children with asthma exposed to high levels of air pollutants. Am J Respir Crit Care Med. Sep 1;166(5):703-9.

80. Trenga CA, Koenig JQ, Williams PV. (2001) Dietary antioxidants and ozone-induced bronchial hyperresponsiveness in adults with asthma. Arch Environ Health. May-Jun;56(3):242-9.

81. Romieu I, et al. (1998) Antioxidant supplementation and respiratory functions among workers exposed to high levels of ozone. Am J Respir Crit Care Med. Jul;158(1):226-32.

82. Grievink L, et al. (1999) Double-blind intervention trial on modulation of ozone effects on pulmonary function by antioxidant supplements. Am J Epidemiol. Feb 15;149(4):306-14.

83. Burbank AJ, et al. (2018) Gamma tocopherol-enriched supplement reduces sputum eosinophilia and endotoxin-induced sputum neutrophilia in volunteers with asthma. *J Allergy Clin Immunol.* Apr;141(4):1231-8.

84. Brehm JM, et al. (2012) Vitamin D insufficiency and severe asthma exacerbations in Puerto Rican children. *Am J Respir Crit Care Med.* Jul 15;186(2):140-6.

85. Brehm JM, et al. (2010) Serum vitamin D levels and severe asthma exacerbations in the Childhood Asthma Management Program study. *J Allergy Clin Immunol.* Jul;126(1):52-8.e5.

86. Brehm JM, et al. (2009) Serum vitamin D levels and markers of severity of childhood asthma in Costa Rica. *Am J Respir Crit Care Med.* May 1;179(9):765-71.

87. Reynolds RD, Natta CL. (1985) Depressed plasma pyridoxal phosphate concentrations in adult asthmatics. *Am J Clin Nutr.* Apr;41(4):684-8.

88. Britton J, et al. (1994) Dietary magnesium, lung function, wheezing, and airway hyperreactivity in a random adult population sample. *Lancet.* Aug 6;344(8919):357-62.

89. Broughton KS, et al. (1997) Reduced asthma symptoms with n-3 fatty acid ingestion are related to 5-series leukotriene production. *Am J Clin Nutr.* Apr;65(4):1011-7.

90. Gupta I, et al. (1998) Effects of Boswellia serrata gum resin in patients with bronchial asthma: results of a double-blind, placebo-controlled, 6-week clinical study. *Eur J Med Res.* Nov 17;3(11):511-4.

91. Potter PC, Klein M, Weinberg EG. (1991) Hydration in severe acute asthma. *Arch Dis Child.* Feb;66(2):216-9.

92. Whyand T, et al. (2018) Pollution and respiratory disease: can diet or supplements help? A review. *Respir Res.* May 2;19(1):79.

93. Bodas M, et al. (2017) Augmentation of S-Nitrosoglutathione Controls Cigarette Smoke-Induced Inflammatory-Oxidative Stress and Chronic Obstructive Pulmonary Disease-Emphysema Pathogenesis by Restoring Cystic Fibrosis Transmembrane Conductance Regulator Function. *Antioxid Redox Signal.* Sep 1;27(7):433-51.

94. Tse HN, et al. (2014) Benefits of high-dose N-acetylcysteine to exacerbation-prone patients with COPD. *Chest.* Sep;146(3):611-23.

95. Zheng JP, et al. (2014) Twice daily N-acetylcysteine 600 mg for exacerbations of chronic obstructive pulmonary disease (PANTHEON): a randomised, double-blind placebo-controlled trial. *Lancet Respir Med.* Mar;2(3):187-94.

Chapter Six References

1. Borre YE, O'Keeffe GW, Clarke G, Stanton C, Dinan TG, Cryan JF. Microbiota and neurodevelopmental windows: implications for brain disorders. *Trends Mol Med.* 2014;20(9):509-518.

2. Maes M, Kubera M, Leunis JC. The gut-brain barrier in major depression: intestinal mucosal dysfunction with an increased translocation of LPS from gram negative enterobacteria (leaky gut) plays a role in the inflammatory pathophysiology of depression. *Neuro Endocrinol Lett.* 2008;29(1):117-124.

3. Fiorentino M, Sapone A, Senger S, et al. Blood-brain barrier and intestinal epithelial barrier alterations in autism spectrum disorders. *Mol Autism.* 2016;7:49.

4. Lochhead JJ, Ronaldson PT, Davis TP. Hypoxic Stress and Inflammatory Pain Disrupt Blood-Brain Barrier Tight Junctions: Implications for Drug Delivery to the Central Nervous System. *Aaps j.* 2017;19(4):910-920.

5. Branton WG, Ellestad KK, Maingat F, et al. Brain microbial populations in HIV/AIDS: α-proteobacteria predominate independent of host immune status. *PLoS One.* 2013;8(1):e54673.

6. Kolappan S, Coureuil M, Yu X, Nassif X, Egelman EH, Craig L. Structure of the Neisseria meningitidis Type IV pilus. *Nat Commun.* 2016;7:13015.

7. Bella R, Lanza G, Cantone M, et al. Effect of a Gluten-Free Diet on Cortical Excitability in Adults with Celiac Disease. *PLoS One.* 2015;10(6):e0129218.

8. Pennisi M, Bramanti A, Cantone M, Pennisi G, Bella R, Lanza G. Neurophysiology of the "Celiac Brain": Disentangling Gut-Brain Connections. *Front Neurosci.* 2017;11:498.

9. Lionetti E, Leonardi S, Franzonello C, Mancardi M, Ruggieri M, Catassi C. Gluten Psychosis: Confirmation of a New Clinical Entity. *Nutrients.* 2015;7(7):5532-5539.

10. Wahab PJ, Crusius JB, Meijer JW, Mulder CJ. Gluten challenge in borderline gluten-sensitive enteropathy. *Am J Gastroenterol.* 2001;96(5):1464-1469.

11. Wikoff WR, Anfora AT, Liu J, et al. Metabolomics analysis reveals large effects of gut microflora on mammalian blood metabolites. *Proc Natl Acad Sci U S A.* 2009;106(10):3698-3703.

12. Yano JM, Yu K, Donaldson GP, et al. Indigenous bacteria from the gut microbiota regulate host serotonin biosynthesis. *Cell.* 2015;161(2):264-276.

13. Samuel BS, Shaito A, Motoike T, et al. Effects of the gut microbiota on host adiposity are modulated by the short-chain fatty-acid binding G protein-coupled receptor, Gpr41. *Proc Natl Acad Sci U S A.* 2008;105(43):16767-16772.

14. Haghikia A, Jörg S, Duscha A, et al. Dietary Fatty Acids Directly Impact Central Nervous System Autoimmunity via the Small Intestine. *Immunity.* 2015;43(4):817-829.

15. Goehler LE, Gaykema RP, Opitz N, Reddaway R, Badr N, Lyte M. Activation in vagal afferents and central autonomic pathways: early responses to intestinal infection with Campylobacter jejuni. *Brain Behav Immun.* 2005;19(4):334-344.

16. Bravo JA, Forsythe P, Chew MV, et al. Ingestion of Lactobacillus strain regulates emotional behavior and central GABA receptor expression in a mouse via the vagus nerve. *Proc Natl Acad Sci U S A.* 2011;108(38):16050-16055.

17. Nayak D, Roth TL, McGavern DB. Microglia development and function. *Annu Rev Immunol.* 2014;32:367-402.

18. Nayak D, Zinselmeyer BH, Corps KN, McGavern DB. In vivo dynamics of innate immune sentinels in the CNS. *Intravital.* 2012;1(2):95-106.

19. Erny D, Hrabě de Angelis AL, Jaitin D, et al. Host microbiota constantly control maturation and function of microglia in the CNS. *Nat Neurosci.* 2015;18(7):965-977.

20. Jessen NA, Munk AS, Lundgaard I, Nedergaard M. The Glymphatic System: A Beginner's Guide. *Neurochem Res.* 2015;40(12):2583-2599.

21. Foster JA, McVey Neufeld KA. Gut-brain axis: how the microbiome influences anxiety and depression. *Trends Neurosci.* 2013;36(5):305-312.

22. Krajmalnik-Brown R, Lozupone C, Kang DW, Adams JB. Gut bacteria in children with autism spectrum disorders: challenges and promise of studying how a complex community influences a complex disease. *Microb Ecol Health Dis.* 2015;26:26914.

23. Severance EG, Yolken RH, Eaton WW. Autoimmune diseases, gastrointestinal disorders and the microbiome in schizophrenia: more than a gut feeling. *Schizophr Res.* 2016;176(1):23-35.

24. Keshavarzian A, Green SJ, Engen PA, et al. Colonic bacterial composition in Parkinson's disease. *Mov Disord.* 2015;30(10):1351-1360.

25. Allnutt MA, Johnson K, Bennett DA, et al. Human Herpesvirus 6 Detection in Alzheimer's Disease Cases and Controls across Multiple Cohorts. *Neuron.* 2020;105(6):1027-1035.e1022.

26. Sweeney MD, Zlokovic BV. A lymphatic waste-disposal system implicated in Alzheimer's disease. *Nature.* 2018;560(7717):172-174.

27. Cermelli C, Berti R, Soldan SS, et al. High frequency of human herpesvirus 6 DNA in multiple sclerosis plaques isolated by laser microdissection. *J Infect Dis.* 2003;187(9):1377-1387.

28. Wipfler P, Dunn N, Beiki O, Trinka E, Fogdell-Hahn A. The Viral Hypothesis of Mesial Temporal Lobe Epilepsy - Is Human Herpes Virus-6 the Missing Link? A systematic review and meta-analysis. *Seizure.* 2018;54:33-40.

Chapter Seven References

1. Segata, N., Boernigen, D., Tickle, T. L., Morgan, X. C., Garrett, W. S., and Huttenhower, C. (2013). Computational metabolomics for microbial community studies. Mol. Syst. Biol. 9:666.

2. Aagaard, K., Petrosino, J., Keitel, W., Watson, M., Katancik, J., Garcia, N., et al. (2013). The Human Microbiome Project strategy for comprehensive sampling of the human microbiome and why it matters. FASEB J. 27, 1012–1022.

3. Lloyd-Price, J., Abu-Ali, G., and Huttenhower, C. (2016). The healthy human microbiome. Genome Med. 8:51.

4. Blekhman, R., Goodrich, J. K., Huang, K., Sun, Q., Bukowski, R., Bell, J. T., et al. (2015). Host genetic variation impacts microbiome composition across human body sites. Genome Biol. 16:191.

5. Vientós-Plotts, A. I., Ericsson, A. C., Rindt, H., Grobman, M. E., Graham, A., Bishop, K., et al. (2017). Dynamic changes of the respiratory microbiota and its relationship to fecal and blood microbiota in healthy young cats. PLoS ONE. 12:e0173818.

6. Mandal, R. K., Jian, T., Al-Rubaye, A. A., Rhoads, D. D., Wideman, R. F., Zhao, J., et al. (2016). An investigation into blood microbiota and its potential association with Bacterial Chondronecrosis with Osteomyelitis (BCO) in broilers. Sci. Rep. 6:25882.

7. Sze, M. A., Tsuruta, M., Yang, S. W., Oh, Y., Man, S. F., Hogg, J. C., et al. (2014). Changes in the bacterial microbiota in gut, blood, and lungs following acute LPS instillation into mice lungs. PLoS ONE 9:e111228.

8. Nikkari, S., McLaughlin, I. J., Bi, W., Dodge, D. E., and Relman, D. A. (2001). Does blood of healthy subjects contain bacterial ribosomal DNA? J. Clin. Microbiol. 39, 1956–1959.

9. McLaughlin, R. W., Vali, H., Lau, P. C., Palfree, R. G., De Ciccio, A., Sirois, M., et al. (2002). Are there naturally occurring pleomorphic bacteria in the blood of healthy humans? J. Clin. Microbiol. 40, 4771–4775.

10. Moriyama, K., Ando, C., Tashiro, K., Kuhara, S., Okamura, S., Nakano, S., et al. (2008). Polymerase chain reaction detection of bacterial 16S rRNA gene in human blood. Microbiol. Immunol. 52, 375–382.

11. Païssé, S., Valle, C., Servant, F., Courtney, M., Burcelin, R., Amar, J., et al. (2016). Comprehensive description of blood microbiome from healthy donors assessed by 16S targeted metagenomic sequencing. Transfusion 56, 1138–1147.

12. de Oliveira C, Watt R, Hamer M. (2010)Toothbrushing, inflammation, and risk of cardiovascular disease: results from Scottish Health Survey. BMJ. May 27;340:c2451.

13. Lockhart, P. B., Brennan, M. T., Sasser, H. C., Fox, P. C., Paster, B. J., & Bahrani-Mougeot, F. K. (2008). Bacteremia Associated with Tooth Brushing and Dental Extraction. Circulation, 117(24), 3118.

14. Potgieter, M., Bester, J., Kell, D. B., and Pretorius, E. (2015). The dormant blood microbiome in chronic, inflammatory diseases. FEMS Microbiol. Rev. 39, 567–591.

15. Dinakaran, V., Rathinavel, A., Pushpanathan, M., Sivakumar, R., Gunasekaran, P., and Rajendhran, J. (2014). Elevated levels of circulating DNA in cardiovascular disease patients:

metagenomic profiling of microbiome in the circulation. PLoS ONE. 9:e105221.

16. Panaiotov, S., Filevski, G., Equestre, M., Nikolova, E., and Kalfin, R. (2018). Cultural isolation and characteristics of the blood microbiome of healthy individuals. Adv. Microbiol. 8:406.

17. Moustafa, A., Xie, C., Kirkness, E., Biggs, W., Wong, E., Turpaz, Y., et al. (2017). The blood DNA virome in 8,000 humans. PLoS Pathog. 13:e1006292.

18. Stremlau, M. H., Andersen, K. G., Folarin, O. A., Grove, J. N., Odia, I., Ehiane, P. E., et al. (2015). Discovery of novel rhabdoviruses in the blood of healthy individuals from West Africa. PLoS Negl. Trop. Dis. 9:e0003631.

19. Rascovan, N., Duraisamy, R., and Desnues, C. (2016). Metagenomics and the human virome in asymptomatic individuals Annu. Rev. Microbiol. 70, 125–141.

20. Furuta, R. A., Sakamoto, H., Kuroishi, A., Yasiui, K., Matsukura, H., and Hirayama, F. (2015). Metagenomic profiling of the viromes of plasma collected from blood donors with elevated serum alanine aminotransferase levels. Transfusion 55, 1889–1899.

21. Aspelund A, Antila S, Proulx ST, Karlsen TV, Karaman S, Detmar M, Wiig H, Alitalo K. (2015) A dural lymphatic vascular system that drains brain interstitial fluid and macromolecules. J Exp Med. Jun 29;212(7):991-9.

22. Louveau A, Smirnov I, Keyes TJ, Eccles JD, Rouhani SJ, Peske JD, Derecki NC, Castle D, Mandell JW, Lee KS, Harris TH, Kipnis J. Structural and functional features of central nervous system

lymphatic vessels. Nature. 2015 Jul 16;523(7560):337-41.

23. Kiernan, M. G., Coffey, J. C., McDermott, K., Cotter, P. D., Cabrera-Rubio, R., Kiely, P. A., & Dunne, C. P. (2019). The Human Mesenteric Lymph Node Microbiome Differentiates Between Crohn's Disease and Ulcerative Colitis. Journal of Crohn's & Colitis, 13(1), 58-66.

24. Funkhouser, L. J., and Bordenstein, S. R. (2013). Mom knows best: the universality of maternal microbial transmission. PLoS Biol. 11:e1001631.

25. Jiménez, E., Fernández, L., Marín, M. L., Martín, R., Odriozola, J. M., Nueno-Palop, C., et al. (2005). Isolation of commensal bacteria from umbilical cord blood of healthy neonates born by cesarean section. Curr. Microbiol. 51, 270–274.

26. Traykova, D., Schneider, B., Chojkier, M., and Buck, M. (2017). Blood microbiome quantity and the hyperdynamic circulation in decompensated cirrhotic patients. PLoS ONE. 12:e0169310.

27. Sato, J., Kanazawa, A., Ikeda, F., Yoshihara, T., Goto, H., Abe, H., et al. (2014). Gut dysbiosis and detection of "live gut bacteria" in blood of Japanese patients with type 2 diabetes. Diabetes Care. 37, 2343–2350.

28. Manzo, V. E., and Bhatt, A. S. (2015). The human microbiome in hematopoiesis and hematologic disorders. Blood 126, 311–318.

29. Morris ZS, Wooding S, Grant J. The answer is 17 years, what is the question: understanding time lags in translational research. J R Soc Med. 2011 Dec;104(12):510-20. doi: 10.1258/jrsm.2011.110180. PMID: 22179294; PMCID: PMC3241518.

Chapter Eight References

1. Gallo RL. Human Skin Is the Largest Epithelial Surface for Interaction with Microbes. *J Invest Dermatol.* 2017;137(6):1213-1214.

2. Verbanic S, Kim CY, Deacon JM, Chen IA. Improved single-swab sample preparation for recovering bacterial and phage DNA from human skin and wound microbiomes. *BMC Microbiol.* 2019;19(1):214.

3. Manrique P, Bolduc B, Walk ST, van der Oost J, de Vos WM, Young MJ. Healthy human gut phageome. *Proc Natl Acad Sci U S A.* 2016;113(37):10400-10405.

4. Probst AJ, Auerbach AK, Moissl-Eichinger C. Archaea on human skin. *PLoS One.* 2013;8(6):e65388.

5. Patra V, Byrne SN, Wolf P. The Skin Microbiome: Is It Affected by UV-induced Immune Suppression? *Front Microbiol.* 2016;7:1235.

6. Cundell AM. Microbial Ecology of the Human Skin. *Microb Ecol.* 2018;76(1):113-120.

7. Grice EA, Kong HH, Conlan S, et al. Topographical and temporal diversity of the human skin microbiome. *Science.* 2009;324(5931):1190-1192.

8. Chloramines in Drinking Water. EPA. https://www.epa.gov/dwreginfo/chloramines-drinking-water. Published 2022. Updated April 18, 2022. Accessed November 22, 2022.

9. B.M. A. *Prevention and Control of Infections in Hospitals: Practice and Theory.* First edition ed. Switzerland: Springer Nature; 2018.

10. Grice EA, Segre JA. The skin microbiome. *Nat Rev Microbiol.* 2011;9(4):244-253.

11. Sherwani MA, Tufail S, Muzaffar AF, Yusuf N. The skin microbiome and immune system: Potential target for chemoprevention? *Photodermatol Photoimmunol Photomed.* 2018;34(1):25-34.

12. Farahmand S. *Skin Microbiome Handbook: From Basic Research to Product Development.* Beverly, MA: Scrivener Publishing LLC; 2020.

13. Bolla BS, Erdei L, Urbán E, Burián K, Kemény L, Szabó K. Cutibacterium acnes regulates the epidermal barrier properties of HPV-KER human immortalized keratinocyte cultures. *Sci Rep.* 2020;10(1):12815.

14. Dimitriu PA, Iker B, Malik K, Leung H, Mohn WW, Hillebrand GG. New Insights into the Intrinsic and Extrinsic Factors That Shape the Human Skin Microbiome. *mBio.* 2019;10(4).

15. Prohic A, Jovovic Sadikovic T, Krupalija-Fazlic M, Kuskunovic-Vlahovljak S. Malassezia species in healthy skin and in dermatological conditions. *Int J Dermatol.* 2016;55(5):494-504.

16. Stehlikova Z, Kostovcik M, Kostovcikova K, et al. Dysbiosis of Skin Microbiota in Psoriatic Patients: Co-occurrence of Fungal and Bacterial Communities. *Front Microbiol.* 2019;10:438.

17. Li M, Budding AE, van der Lugt-Degen M, Du-Thumm L, Vandeven M, Fan A. The influence of age, gender and race/ethnicity on the composition of the human axillary microbiome. *Int J Cosmet Sci.* 2019;41(4):371-377.

18. Ying S, Zeng DN, Chi L, et al. The Influence of Age and Gender on Skin-Associated Microbial Communities in Urban and Rural Human Populations. *PLoS One.* 2015;10(10):e0141842.

19. Ehlers C, Ivens UI, Møller ML, Senderovitz T, Serup J. Females have lower skin surface pH than men. A study on the surface of gender, forearm site variation, right/left difference and time of the day on the skin surface pH. *Skin Res Technol.* 2001;7(2):90-94.

20. Levy G. The Human Microbiome and Gender Medicine. *Gender Genome.* 2018;2:123.

21. Edmonds-Wilson SL, Nurinova NI, Zapka CA, Fierer N, Wilson M. Review of human hand microbiome research. *J Dermatol Sci.* 2015;80(1):3-12.

22. Flak MB, Neves JF, Blumberg RS. Immunology. Welcome to the microgenderome. *Science.* 2013;339(6123):1044-1045.

23. Kwok YL, Gralton J, McLaws ML. Face touching: a frequent habit that has implications for hand hygiene. *Am J Infect Control.* 2015;43(2):112-114.

24. Hospodsky D, Pickering AJ, Julian TR, et al. Hand bacterial communities vary across two different human populations. *Microbiology (Reading).* 2014;160(Pt 6):1144-1152.

25. Xu H, Li H. Acne, the Skin Microbiome, and Antibiotic Treatment. *Am J Clin Dermatol.* 2019;20(3):335-344.

26. Sardana K, Gupta T, Kumar B, Gautam HK, Garg VK. Cross-sectional Pilot Study of Antibiotic Resistance in Propionibacterium Acnes Strains in Indian Acne Patients Using 16S-RNA Polymerase Chain Reaction: A Comparison Among Treatment Modalities Including Antibiotics, Benzoyl

Peroxide, and Isotretinoin. *Indian J Dermatol.* 2016;61(1):45-52.

27. Chien AL, Tsai J, Leung S, et al. Association of Systemic Antibiotic Treatment of Acne With Skin Microbiota Characteristics. *JAMA Dermatol.* 2019;155(4):425-434.

28. Park SY, Kim HS, Lee SH, Kim S. Characterization and Analysis of the Skin Microbiota in Acne: Impact of Systemic Antibiotics. *J Clin Med.* 2020;9(1).

29. Callewaert C, Knödlseder N, Karoglan A, Güell M, Paetzold B. Skin microbiome transplantation and manipulation: Current state of the art. *Comput Struct Biotechnol J.* 2021;19:624-631.

30. Costello EK, Lauber CL, Hamady M, Fierer N, Gordon JI, Knight R. Bacterial community variation in human body habitats across space and time. *Science.* 2009;326(5960):1694-1697.

31. Perin B, Addetia A, Qin X. Transfer of skin microbiota between two dissimilar autologous microenvironments: A pilot study. *PLoS One.* 2019;14(12):e0226857.

32. Myles IA, Earland NJ, Anderson ED, et al. First-in-human topical microbiome transplantation with Roseomonas mucosa for atopic dermatitis. *JCI Insight.* 2018;3(9).

Chapter Nine References

1. Gustafson C. Bruce Ames, phd, and Rhonda Patrick, phd: Discussing the Triage Concept and the Vitamin D-Serotonin Connection. *IMCJ*. 2014;13(6):34-42.

2. Shelor CP, Kirk AB, Dasgupta PK, Kroll M, Campbell CA, Choudhary PK. Breastfed infants metabolize perchlorate. *Environ Sci Technol*. 2012;46(9):5151-5159.

3. Cho KM, Math RK, Islam SM, et al. Biodegradation of chlorpyrifos by lactic acid bacteria during kimchi fermentation. *J Agric Food Chem*. 2009;57(5):1882-1889.

4. Islam SM, Math RK, Cho KM, et al. Organophosphorus hydrolase (OpdB) of Lactobacillus brevis WCP902 from kimchi is able to degrade organophosphorus pesticides. *J Agric Food Chem*. 2010;58(9):5380-5386.

5. Oishi K, Sato T, Yokoi W, Yoshida Y, Ito M, Sawada H. Effect of probiotics, Bifidobacterium breve and Lactobacillus casei, on bisphenol A exposure in rats. *Biosci Biotechnol Biochem*. 2008;72(6):1409-1415.

6. Ebrahimi M, Khalili N, Razi S, Keshavarz-Fathi M, Khalili N, Rezaei N. Effects of lead and cadmium on the immune system and cancer progression. *J Environ Health Sci Eng*. 2020;18(1):335-343.

7. Assefa S, Köhler G. Intestinal Microbiome and Metal Toxicity. *Curr Opin Toxicol*. 2020;19:21-27.

8. Chen Z, Tang Z, Kong J, et al. Lactobacillus casei SYF-08 Protects Against Pb-Induced Injury in Young Mice by Regulating Bile Acid Metabolism and Increasing Pb Excretion. *Front Nutr*. 2022;9:914323.

9. Zhai Q, Liu Y, Wang C, et al. Lactobacillus plantarum CCFM8661 modulates bile acid enterohepatic circulation and increases lead excretion in mice. *Food Funct.* 2019;10(3):1455-1464.

10. Zhai Q, Liu Y, Wang C, et al. Increased Cadmium Excretion Due to Oral Administration of Lactobacillus plantarum Strains by Regulating Enterohepatic Circulation in Mice. *J Agric Food Chem.* 2019;67(14):3956-3965.

11. Zhai Q, Tian F, Zhao J, Zhang H, Narbad A, Chen W. Oral Administration of Probiotics Inhibits Absorption of the Heavy Metal Cadmium by Protecting the Intestinal Barrier. *Appl Environ Microbiol.* 2016;82(14):4429-4440.

12. Mullenix PJ. A new perspective on metals and other contaminants in fluoridation chemicals. *Int J Occup Environ Health.* 2014;20(2):157-166.

13. Laparra JM, Sanz Y. Bifidobacteria inhibit the inflammatory response induced by gliadins in intestinal epithelial cells via modifications of toxic peptide generation during digestion. *J Cell Biochem.* 2010;109(4):801-807.

14. Helmerhorst EJ, Zamakhchari M, Schuppan D, Oppenheim FG. Discovery of a novel and rich source of gluten-degrading microbial enzymes in the oral cavity. *PLoS One.* 2010;5(10):e13264.

15. Endo H, Higurashi T, Hosono K, et al. Efficacy of Lactobacillus casei treatment on small bowel injury in chronic low-dose aspirin users: a pilot randomized controlled study. *J Gastroenterol.* 2011;46(7):894-905.

16. Oh CK, Oh MC, Kim SH. The depletion of sodium nitrite by lactic acid bacteria isolated from kimchi. *J Med Food.* 2004;7(1):38-44.

17. Tan M, Zhu JC, Du J, Zhang LM, Yin HH. Effects of probiotics on serum levels of Th1/Th2 cytokine and clinical outcomes in severe traumatic brain-injured patients: a prospective randomized pilot study. *Crit Care.* 2011;15(6):R290.

18. Wada M, Nagata S, Saito M, et al. Effects of the enteral administration of Bifidobacterium breve on patients undergoing chemotherapy for pediatric malignancies. *Support Care Cancer.* 2010;18(6):751-759.

19. Environmental Health Symposium https://www.environmentalhealthsymposium.com/ Accessed.

20. Turnbaugh PJ, Ley RE, Hamady M, Fraser-Liggett CM, Knight R, Gordon JI. The human microbiome project. *Nature.* 2007;449(7164):804-810.

21. AM K. *Peptide Immunotherapy: COLOSTUM, A Physician's Reference Guide.* AKS Publishing2009.

22. Inglot AD, Janusz M, Lisowski J. Colostrinine: a proline-rich polypeptide from ovine colostrum is a modest cytokine inducer in human leukocytes. *Arch Immunol Ther Exp (Warsz).* 1996;44(4):215-224.

23. Pang, S., Chen, X., Lu, Z. *et al.* Longevity of centenarians is reflected by the gut microbiome with youth-associated signatures. *Nat Aging* (2023). https://doi.org/10.1038/s43587-023-00389-y

24. Crinnion, WH. Private memorandum; Oct 2019

Made in the USA
Middletown, DE
07 November 2023

42096394R00144